Asperger Syndrome & Your Child

Asperger Syndrome & Your Child

A PARENT'S GUIDE

Michael D. Powers, Psy.D.

with Janet Poland

A SKYLIGHT PRESS BOOK

Consulting Editor, Denise Grenier

HarperResource

An Imprint of HarperCollins*Publishers*

Grateful acknowledgment is made to the publishers and individuals for permission to use the following text: An adaptation of "Educator's Compassion Takes on Expert's Statistics on Autism" by Michael Bernick from the *San Francisco Chronicle*, January 27, 2002: Reprinted by permission of the author. An adaptation of pages 340–366 from *Asperger Syndrome* by Ami Klin and Fred Volkmar: Reprinted by permission of the Guilford Press. An adaptation of "Understanding the Student with Asperger Syndrome; Guidelines for Teachers" by Karen Williams. Reprinted with permission, June 1995, *Focus in Autistic Behavior, Vol. 10,* 9–16. Copyright 1995 by PRO-ED. An adaptation of the social conversation checklist from *Work in Progress* by John McEachin and Ronald Leaf: Reprinted by permission of Autism Partnership. "The Letter I Never Wrote My Parents" by Jerry Newport: Reprinted by permission of Future Horizons.

HarperCollins books may be purchased for educational, business, or sales promotional use. For information please write: Special Markets Department, HarperCollins Publishers Inc., 10 East 53rd Street, New York, NY 10022.

FIRST EDITION

Designed by William Ruoto

Library of Congress Cataloging-in-Publication Data

Powers, Michael D.
Asperger syndrome and your child: a parent's guide/[Michael D. Powers, Janet Poland].
p.cm.
Includes bibliographical references.
ISBN 0-06-620943-9
1. Asperger's syndrome—Popular works. I. Poland, Janet. II. Title.
RJ506.A9 P69 2002
618.92'8982—dc21
2002190234

04 05 06 ❖/QWM 10 9 8 7 6 5 4 3 2

For Kristen, Seth, Evan, and Kaden

Contents

Acknowledgments

As much as this book is *about* Asperger Syndrome, it is also about *living* with Asperger Syndrome. I have been very fortunate to have many exceptional teachers on this subject, especially the parents and families with whom I have worked over the past twenty-five years. They have contributed their stories about their hopes, fears, and dreams for their children to my work and life, enriching me in ways too numerous to recount.

I have been privileged to know Temple Grandin and Jerry Newport for many years, and have been enriched by their keen, often frank observations about their lives and the world we "neurotypicals" present to them. I am indebted to them for all that they have taught me.

Liane Holliday Willey, through her wonderful books and lectures, brought a remarkable perspective to my understanding of Asperger Syndrome. By so eloquently describing both her own and her daughters' struggles and triumphs with this condition, Liane reminds us all that we are mothers and fathers, brothers, sisters, and children first and foremost. Those differences that make us unique can empower all those around us, if only we allow it.

Jerry Newport's "The Letter I Never Wrote My Parents" appeared originally in the *Autism/Asperger Digest*. It is one of the most strikingly poignant and honest pieces of writing in our field, and Jerry graciously has allowed me to reprint it here. With his characteristic sense of irony and humor, Jerry addresses a question asked of me by so many parents: "What will become of my child?" Jerry's ability to put his life into words—and perspective—reinforces a central theme of this book: All lives well lived have hopes, dreams, and travails, but the ability to grow, understand, and look at one's life with satisfaction overall requires an appreciation of the ups and downs. It is what makes us whole, and allows others to be ennobled by our experiences. Thank you, Jerry, for the privilege of reprinting your work.

Michael Bernick's article on his son Will's experiences with a community basketball team first appeared in the *San Francisco Chronicle*, and is excerpted in chapter 6, "The Wedged and the Winners." By reminding us that inclusion is all about starting out at the level of the child's abilities, this father highlights the positive effect of that understanding on classmates and peers without disabilities. Thank you, Michael, for permission to include this wonderful story.

Evan Powers and several of his close friends, working together with students in Barnstable, Massachusetts, created the "Tips for Being a Friend" reprinted in chapter 8. Thanks to each of them for providing a kid's eye view of this most important area. As a clinician, I am always amazed by the wisdom and thoughtfulness of children who, if only offered the chance, will reach out to classmates with special needs. As a father, I am privileged to be in the constant company of one such student.

Drs. Ami Klin, Fred Volkmar, and Sara Sparrow, my colleagues at the Yale Child Study Center, have graciously permitted me to adapt material on appropriate educational settings from their outstanding book *Asperger Syndrome* (Guilford Press, 2000). For this, for their friendship, and for their many efforts on behalf of those with Asperger Syndrome and their families, I am grateful.

Several years ago I came upon an article written by Karen Williams, of the University of Michigan Medical Center Child and Adolescent Psychiatric Hospital, on strategies for teaching students with Asperger Syndrome. Since the publication of this article in *Focus on Autistic Behavior*, I have reviewed many other papers on similar topics, all valuable. Few, however, address these critical issues with the parsimony and straightforward tone of Williams's work. I appreciate Karen's willingness to allow me to disseminate these strategies to an even wider audience.

The world of Asperger Syndrome would not be what it is today without OASIS, the award-winning Web site (www.aspergersyndrome.org) created by Barbara Kirby. As an online resource for parents and professionals, it is without parallel. The new *OASIS Guide to Asperger Syndrome* (Crown, 2001) is yet another remarkable product of the creative energies of coauthors Patricia Romanowski Bashe and Barbara Kirby. If information is power, then OASIS is the sun. Thank you, Barbara, for all that you have done.

Dawn Barrett and Liz Noble at our Center for Children with Special Needs provided exceptional support in the preparation of this manuscript. Their efforts on this project, as with all others, are deeply appreciated.

Many thanks, also, to Dania Jekel of the Asperger's Association of New England for her valuable insights, to Marcy Hynes for illuminating the classroom experiences of children with Asperger Syndrome and their teachers, and to Deborah Cervas, who provided the social story in chapter 8. And a heartfelt thanks to the adults and children with Asperger Syndrome and their families, who prefer to remain anonymous, but who have helped make this book what it is.

I have been fortunate indeed to work with editors at Skylight Press and HarperCollins who have provided thoughtful guidance, a refined and critical eye, and encouragement throughout the preparation of this book. To Lynn Sonberg, Meg Schneider, and Denise Grenier at Skylight and to Megan Newman and Kathryn Huck at HarperCollins, I owe many thanks.

Beyond her role as consulting editor for Skylight Press, Denise Grenier contributed many examples, thoughtful comments, and a seasoned parental perspective to this book. If the clinical and case examples provide the heart and soul of *Asperger Syndrome and Your Child,* then Denise's many contributions nurtured that effort immeasurably. Thank you, Denise.

Joe, Cindy, and Anthony Varrone and Tony and Ann Dellorfano have been among my finest teachers on the power of family in a child's life. They have welcomed our family into theirs, sharing the delight and celebration of their son's and grandson's achievements. I am indebted to them for their friendship and for the wonderful example they provide.

Dr. Sandra Harris has been my guiding spirit and mentor in my work in autism spectrum disorders for over twenty years. As a teacher, she is without parallel. As a friend, she is one of life's finest gifts.

Without question, this book would not exist without Janet Poland. She has been the consummate collaborator, weaving prose from outlines and notes. From working and reworking the manuscript through countless drafts and queries, to helping me stay on schedule (more than anyone else has ever been able to do), Janet's keen eye for the written word, good humor, and unrelenting patience have made the process of creating this book together a delight.

Finally, it is for my family that my most heartfelt gratitude is reserved. To my wonderful sons Seth, Evan, and Kaden: You never fail to remind me of what is most precious in life, and that it is the journey—not the destination—that matters most.

And for my wife, Kristen, who so effortlessly combines the role of partner, parent, and professional colleague, I can only say with love:

"More is thy due than more than all can pay."
(Shakespeare, Macbeth, Act 1, Scene 4, line 21)

Foreword

Knowledge of Asperger Syndrome comes to the scientific community like seasonal showers come to parched roads. News and information don't appear in great deluges, ready to overwhelm and fill each nook and cranny of our need to know, our need to understand, and our need to help. Rather, tiny drops of information fall in slapdash style, bringing only a subtle amount of relief to a community with seemingly endless questions and never enough answers. Like so many families affected by Asperger Syndrome, I know precisely how it feels to sit in doctors' waiting rooms and counselors' offices and school administrators' meetings, hoping and praying for a soaking shower of solidly helpful information that will serve to make my family's life with AS fresh and quenched. Dr. Michael Powers's book answers those hopes and those prayers. His book is a brilliant rain!

I have often read books on AS that do much to share credible research and good information, but very rarely have I read a book that strikes the chords of insight and accuracy as strongly as Dr. Powers's book does. Dr. Powers understands what AS is, not just in a clinical manner, but in a human way. His words are honest and direct, but filled with compassion and empathy for the people I am fortunate enough to call my peers: the people with AS. Yet, never does the empathy and compassion turn into condescension or disrespect. There always remains a deeply hued richness that serves to paint a strikingly vivid picture of what AS truly is, from its marrow to its surreal. In brilliant style, Dr. Powers weaves together an extremely comprehensive and easy-to-read account of everything conceivably related to AS.

Who should read this book? My quick answer is everyone, for the book is that important to our society as a whole. But more specifically, I will say that all who seek to understand the gifts and the pathos, as well as the exuberance and the struggles, that come to one with an atypical neurosystem should definitely add this book to their world. Parents, caretakers, counselors, and medical professionals—every one could benefit from the insight Dr. Powers provides. And so, too, will people personally affected with AS. It is often difficult to read what others have to say about "my population." My skin tends to stretch a bit too tightly when I read what some *think* we with AS are thinking and feeling and needing. My skin felt just fine when I read *Asperger Syndrome and Your Child*. In fact, it felt great.

I am proud to recommend this book to those who want and need to know about AS. I can honestly say this book will give you the most highly respected bits of research, the clearest ideas, and the most sound advice on intervention and support. And in so doing, this book will open hearts, soothe broken spirits, encourage new dreams, and clear the path for what we all long for and deserve: mutual respect and appreciation.

Thank you, Dr. Powers, for writing a book I could trust my heart to.

—Liane Holliday Willey, Ed.D., author of *Pretending to Be Normal: Living with Asperger's Syndrome* and *Asperger Syndrome in the Family: Redefining Normal*

Introduction

Asperger Syndrome has a short history but a long past. From the astute observations of Dr. Hans Asperger in the years preceding his 1944 publication of *Die "Autistischen Psychopathen" im Kindesalter,* to the proliferation of reports and descriptions of Asperger Syndrome in the popular press and scientific literature, we find ourselves today in the midst of an information explosion about a condition few knew existed twenty years ago.

Some writers have suggested that certain enigmatic creative historical figures, from Thomas Jefferson to Albert Einstein, as well as certain present-day captains of commerce, might be diagnosed with Asperger Syndrome. This diagnostic sleuthing—whether valid or not—is an understandable effort to make sense of people who appear so similar to us in some ways, but are also different in inexplicable ways. From this perspective, this book is an attempt to further that effort, to examine the ways in which we are the same, as well as different, and to place Asperger Syndrome within the fascinating spectrum of human variation.

My own clinical career with individuals with Asperger Syndrome has incorporated experiences as a special education teacher, psychologist, university faculty member, therapist, and program consultant. I have worked both in the United States and abroad with parents, classroom teachers from primary through university levels, a wide variety of health care professionals, and—most importantly—individuals with Asperger Syndrome themselves in numerous settings. My understanding and appreciation of those with Asperger Syndrome are based on those experiences, and serve as the basis for blending scientific and clinical perspectives on this enigmatic condition in order to promote a better understanding and awareness for parents and professionals.

When we first began to plan and write *Asperger Syndrome and Your Child,* there were fewer than five published books available on Asperger Syndrome. Recently, books describing current scientific findings, resources for families and professionals, and many first-person accounts have become available, enlarging our understanding immensely. In our book we seek to add yet another layer of understanding, namely a clinician's view of Asperger Syndrome derived from work with children, adolescents, adults, and their families.

We believe this perspective is important for several reasons. Unlike many individuals with autism and other developmental disorders, people with Asperger Syndrome are often highly capable of sharing their experiences with us. So we have a unique opportunity to listen to and learn from the real experts—those with the condition itself. Thus, our understanding of this condition can go beyond the scientific observation and characterization of symptoms and enter the real world in which people live.

We can learn from them, as well as from scientific observation, what it is like to grow up in a family, in a community, in a school, and what it takes to forge a career and establish a satisfying relationship. For people with Asperger Syndrome and their families, that crucial harmony of temperament, often called "goodness of fit" (or the absence of it), often defines the quality of an experience; we can learn from them what settings, which accommodations, what interventions make life go more smoothly, and which do not.

Asperger Syndrome and Your Child was written for parents and professionals as an introduction to this remarkable and complex condition. We have attempted to provide a balanced, informative view of those with Asperger Syndrome enhanced by the stories of children, adolescents, and adults and their families, about their triumphs and challenges facing a world ill-prepared to understand their uniqueness and gifts. (Although these stories are true, names and identifying details have been changed, except where noted, to protect privacy.)

Although more boys than girls are diagnosed with Asperger Syndrome, we use "he" and "she" pronouns equally, alternating by chapter. We hope that *Asperger Syndrome and Your Child* will be the start of a comprehensive, informative, hopeful, exhilarating journey for those who live and work with those with the condition.

The book is divided into two sections. Part I summarizes what we know about Asperger Syndrome in fairly general terms and takes you on a guided tour of the mind of the child with this syndrome. We discuss what scientists believe is different about the brain in people with this disorder, and then hear from people with Asperger Syndrome about how they perceive the world and their place in it, and what approaches they feel have helped them in school, in the community, and in their social lives.

We discuss the important topic of diagnosis, taking parents step-by-step from earliest observation of symptoms through evaluation, testing, and finally, a diagnosis. We then turn to the issue of how parents can expect to feel once the diagnosis is confirmed, and how to share this information with others.

In Part II, we talk about how to apply what we know about Asperger Syndrome to the unique circumstances of your own child within your own family and community. We explore the impact of this disorder on the entire family, including other siblings; offer practical suggestions on how to structure family life to provide an environment that is both secure and stimulating; and discuss how to manage your child's behavior and develop reasonable rules and expectations. We follow your child out the door into the community, focusing on ways to help your child develop the skills that will be needed as he or she moves from the safe haven of family. Practical matters like greeting neighbors, going to an amusement park, and going on play dates are addressed, as is the issue of how to manage—and help your child manage—unusual behaviors and anxieties in public or social settings.

Then in chapter 7 we discuss the crucial elementary school years, the years during which Asperger Syndrome makes its greatest impact on families as children may exhibit anxieties, have trouble with certain academic areas and social relationships, and run into unsympathetic peers and teachers. An essential part of this chapter describes how to request and demand appropriate school services for your child, and how to provide a nurturing and secure home environment. We include a brief guide designed specifically for you to share with your child's teacher.

We also examine the social aspects of your child's school years, and outline practical techniques that have helped many children with Asperger Syndrome improve their skills; make friends; and enjoy social, athletic, and group activities.

Later, we approach the process of leaving the nest and finding one's place among one's peers. This is the crucial task of adolescence, but young people with Asperger Syndrome have a particularly difficult time taking these steps. We examine how parents can help their children hone social skills, build self-confidence, learn independence and personal security, and make educational and career decisions.

Finally, the last chapter focuses on ways to help older adolescents work toward independence and examines the prognosis for successful lives for adults with Asperger Syndrome. Many such young people are coping well, and this chapter shares their stories with you and your child.

Asperger Syndrome remains something of a mystery. There's much we have yet to learn. Yet there is so much we have learned, especially about what approaches and techniques are effective in helping children with Asperger Syndrome become their finest selves.

The time has come to pull together what we know about Asperger Syndrome, the therapies and techniques we know to be effective in real children, and the strategies that we know can help real families who need help now.

Part One

Understanding
Asperger Syndrome

1

Maps, Globes, Continents, and Seas

What Does Asperger Syndrome Look Like?

"My name is not Brendan. My name is Zimbabwe."

So began my interview with a lively, charming five-year-old.

"It's not my real name, you know. It's my pretend name that I like because Zimbabwe is such a beautiful country. Dr. Powers, do you know about continents?"

During the next three hours I learned which countries in Africa bordered Zimbabwe, the capitals of each, and the names of these regions during the time of European control. I learned about the difference between seas and oceans, a condensed explanation of tectonic plates, and the origin of the Mercator projection. I also learned about the strategies a little boy used to organize his world and his determined (but often unsuccessful) efforts to engage his peers with his knowledge and interests.

From precocious beginnings, Brendan had always been somewhat of an enigma. He was an early talker. He surprised his parents by reading "octagon" at age two. He quickly established himself as a wunderkind (or was it whirling dervish?) by three. He could see a picture on a Legos box and build it effortlessly. He remembered not only the names of his parents' friends' siblings, but also the type of car they drove.

Given a topic that caught his interest, he would amass facts and information. His topic branched quickly. Building Legos became an interest in vehicles, which begot an interest in airplanes, which begot propellers, which became his interest in wind currents around the globe. After a while no one was very surprised by a topic or fact that Brendan might introduce into a conversation.

Except the other children in kindergarten. They were never sure about what to expect from Brendan. He was pleasant enough, although somewhat standoffish. Well-behaved, but a bit temperamental sometimes, like the day the class was studying the number 100, and Brendan was going to bring in his collection of flags from countries around the world and distribute them among the children in groups of ten. Problem was, he had 141 flags, and despaired about which he might have to exclude to make it all come out even. His distress was evident to his classmates from the moment he entered the room. Brendan's tearful, often breathless description of his dilemma to his teacher confused some children and mildly frightened others. His rigidity and unpredictability made it hard for the other children to make friends with him.

Looking back, Brendan's parents laugh when recalling the names he has selected for himself over the years. Once, when memorizing the fifty states and capitals, he selected Wyoming for his new name and became indignant when his parents called him by his birth name.

Brendan's parents theorize that he selected Wyoming and Zimbabwe as his names because they were last on the lists he had memorized in alphabetical order. But Brendan disagrees, insisting that he selected them because he likes the sounds of the words and because both are beautiful places.

In my efforts to understand this little boy, I am struck by the elegant simplicity of his assertion. The symbolism we attach to ourselves may be utterly personal, and often misunderstood. But it is no less special, and no less worthy of understanding by others. Recognizing Brendan's true self, and his right to that self, will be our challenge as we help him develop his gifts and share them with others.

And that is our challenge as we try to understand and appreciate the Brendans of the world. Whether we are their mothers or fathers or teachers or neighbors or favorite aunts, we and they will flourish when we learn as much as we can about the sometimes heartbreaking, sometimes exhilarating, condition known as Asperger Syndrome.

Many children with this disability grow up to lead full lives—having careers, bringing joy to their families, and sometimes marrying. Others may lead quite restricted lives. Much depends on the degree to which they have learned to cope with the difficulties that the condition brings. There is a great deal we can do to help children with Asperger Syndrome bring their remarkable gifts to fruition, and in my years of experience working with children with developmental disorders, I have learned much about what parents can do that works well and what doesn't work so well.

The fall of 1976 provided me with my first clear experience of the paradox of Asperger Syndrome. While I had worked with children with autism at Rutgers University several years earlier, my first job as a special education teacher of seventh and eighth graders in New Jersey introduced me to Phillip.

Phillip was brilliant, yet confusing. He was shy and remote most of the time, except when delving into his current passion, usually about animals. At those times, he brightened, smiled, and welcomed me (and anyone else who would listen) into his world. My interest was piqued. I spent the next two years as Phillip's teacher, and also as his pupil.

Some twenty-five years later, the world I learned about from Phillip and many others holds an even greater fascination for me than when I began my studies in that junior high classroom. Through their stories, experiences, travails, and triumphs, the people with Asperger Syndrome whom I have known have taught me more about diversity, culture, courage, and the quirkiness of the world than I could ever have learned on my own. I will always be in their debt.

The Defining Traits
of Asperger Syndrome

Asperger Syndrome (also called Asperger Disorder) is a neurological condition that affects social and emotional interaction. It is a developmental disability, which means that it is most likely present at birth and affects development throughout life.

The four essential qualities that characterize children with Asperger Syndrome are significant difficulties with social interactions, impaired communication, unusual or unusually rigid behaviors and interests, and unusual responses to stimulation and environment. Let's begin with the most important of the four.

Impaired Social Interaction. Six-year-old Sean, on meeting a new child at school, opened the conversation this way: "Did you know that Mars is a 4.5-billion-year-old planet? And although most people think it's red, it's really yellow and brown. In 1976, the *Viking 2* lander took color pictures...." Sean continued to spout facts about Mars, oblivious to the other child's rapidly declining interest.

Children with Asperger Syndrome may not appear unusual until they reach the preschool years, during which children broaden their social worlds, learn to socialize in a group, and forge friendships. At this stage, it becomes more evident that they are having difficulty learning the nonverbal and subtle aspects of social interaction that most children seem to learn effortlessly; they may not recognize the meaning and cues that come from other people's facial expressions or gestures or body language.

Children with Asperger Syndrome have difficulty learning the social graces that most children learn intuitively, although all children make errors as they learn. The easy give and take of play may be a mystery to children with Asperger Syndrome. Ben, a seven-year-old, was often invited to friends' houses for play dates, but he was never invited back. His mystified mother asked around until she learned that Ben's procedure, on arriving at the friend's house, was to collect an armful of books and retire to the bathroom, where he would read for the remainder of the time.

As children grow older, they may learn social rules but apply them improperly. They often are eager to establish social connections, but misuse the lessons they have learned about etiquette or social behavior, or may become too rigid and legalistic in their interpretations. They may be perceived as tattletales, for their persistence in pointing out rule violations in others. They may become sticklers for accuracy at inappropriate times.

Rashid, for example, got into a scuffle with another child in their fourth-grade classroom, and hit him with a book. When the teacher intervened, a witness stated that Rashid had hit the other boy "with an atlas." Rashid objected, saying, "Excuse me, but that is not correct. It was not an atlas, but an official 1977 Almanac, second edition." Rashid did not realize that his statement not only was irrelevant, but did not in the least help his case.

Impaired Communication. Unlike children with autism, who often develop only limited language, children with Asperger Syndrome frequently learn language skills early, often precociously. Eric, for example, was an early talker and developed an extensive vocabulary. His parents and other adults were impressed, but his playmates began to find him off-putting. In the elementary school cafeteria, for example, Eric spilled a bowl of applesauce. The other kids laughed and teased him good-naturedly. Eric replied, "It's not my fault. You startled me, making me jerk involuntarily, and create this unsightly mess."

Many bright children, of course, are early talkers, learn their letters early, and pick up mature speech patterns from their elders. What is different about children with Asperger Syndrome, however, is in the way these skills are applied.

The social application of language is called pragmatics. How to make small talk, how to take turns in conversation, how to change the subject gracefully, all are skills that most people learn early in life and refine over time. As we will discuss in the following chapter, these seemingly natural abilities are linked intimately with the development of particular regions of the brain, and with the brain's ability to organize information in certain ways.

Children with Asperger Syndrome have great difficulty mastering these often unspoken rules of communication. They may monopolize a conversation, or they may use a social interaction as an opportunity to expound on their favorite topic. They may be unable to switch topics easily, a skill that makes casual social discourse possible. Or they may switch unpredictably from topic to topic, confusing their conversational partners.

The difficulty that children with Asperger Syndrome have in gauging the point of view of other people makes conversation even more difficult. Most of us, when we chat with someone, intuitively adjust our comments to our partner's needs. We provide background information as we go along. We pick up cues from our conversational partner—a nod and smile, for example, tell us that we've been understood, a furrowed brow tells us we need to provide a bit more detail.

People with Asperger Syndrome have great difficulty in making these adjustments. They may plunge ahead with their topics and ignore cues from the other speaker. It may not dawn on them that the other person has no interest in the subject, although this skill can be learned. I remember sitting at dinner with a colleague with Asperger Syndrome at a conference we had given together. He pointed out to those at the table the five-blade ceiling fan overhead. After asking us if we knew the difference in air volume moved between a four-blade and five-blade fan, he commented that maybe we didn't want to know that much about the fan, but rather cared only whether it worked. He then suggested another topic.

All children may commit conversational faux pas from time to time, of course. But generally, typical kids refine their skills with practice and maturity. Children with Asperger Syndrome have difficulty learning these skills intuitively, so they'll benefit from the techniques we outline for developing conversational and social skills.

Repetitive or Odd Patterns of Behavior or Interests. Like Brendan and his maps, children with Asperger Syndrome often demonstrate a preoccupation with a narrow interest or unusual topic. Generally, these interests result in huge collections of facts and memorized bits of information, but little generalized context. Thus, as we discussed above, these children often approach others with lists and recitations about subjects, rather than with more acceptable social icebreakers.

It is important to distinguish between the intense and focused interests that many children have, and the relentless focus of the child with Asperger Syndrome. Many children collect facts about Mars, or dinosaurs, or have a voracious interest in jet airplanes. But the child with Asperger Syndrome is different, because the focus is oddly limited. It's as though the facts are gathered and treasured like little jewels, rather than as part of a cohesive subject that broadens as more information is acquired.

A child who collects baseball cards may obsessively memorize the statistics and uniform numbers, but also show some interest in the game of baseball and the social aspects of collecting and trading the cards. The child with Asperger Syndrome not only memorizes and recites endless statistics, but may zero in on less relevant details, such as the intricacies of each team's uniform, and use this knowledge in an off-putting way, rather than as an entrée into social experiences.

Sometimes, the behavior is expressed through ritual behavior, and a need for sameness that the child may cling to as a lifeline. Any deviation from past behavior is profoundly upsetting. Each time Ramon was taken shopping for snow boots, for example, he insisted on the same style and color. Year after year he'd get the same boots, but in a larger size. The crisis came when he outgrew the children's section, and found no such boots were available in the men's section. His parents were mortified as he grabbed the child-size boots and tried to stuff his big feet into them. He became so upset that they had to leave the store without boots.

Unusual Responses to Stimulation and Environment. Andrew appears distracted in class. When his teacher asks what he is doing, he replies that he is listening to the voices. The teacher worries that Andrew may be suffering from hallucinations and refers him to the school psychologist who discovers that he was listening to real voices in the hall, which no one else in the classroom could hear.

It is not unusual for children with Asperger Syndrome to have acute senses of smell, hearing, or taste. Ironically, sometimes the very acuity of the senses makes the child appear impaired; some children appear to be hearing-impaired because they become so focused on a subtle sound that they block out, and become unresponsive to, other sounds and voices.

In some cases, the senses themselves may be normal, but the child's emotional response to stimuli may be heightened. Seven-year-old Laura had what her parents thought were nightmares, often waking up screaming about earthquakes. What upset Laura turned out to be the vibration from the washing machine spin cycle, which in Laura's sleepy state felt like threatening earth tremors.

Often, the child experiences a negative response to the sheer volume of sensory input, whether it is bright light, loud noises, or strong odors. Such children may shy away from activities that everyone assumes all children enjoy: recess, with its noise and unpredictable movements, or amusement parks and carnival rides. One otherwise athletic child refused to participate in track meets because he found the crack of the starter pistol excruciating.

Often, however, troublesome responses to stimuli are harder to explain. For some, it's the hum of a fluorescent light that irritates; for others, it's the buzz of the fire drill alarm. These sounds may prompt an emotional response—from mild agitation to a full-fledged tantrum—

that appears out of proportion to any discomfort the child might be experiencing.

Also typical of Asperger Syndrome is a tendency in some children to move in an ungainly or repetitive manner. The child may walk on tiptoes, flap the hands at the wrists, and exhibit fidgeting, twitches, or tics.

Of course, many children are sensitive to sensory stimuli, tend to fidget, and have trouble with transitions or sudden changes in routine. In Asperger Syndrome, however, these sensitivities combine with the core traits of social and communicative impairment.

It's also important to note that children with Asperger Syndrome may have a greater risk than other children for depression or anxiety. Clearly, when the environment seems threatening, and the social environment is mystifying, a child feels anxious. Older children, in particular, may be painfully aware of their isolation, and be prone to depression.

Often, children with Asperger Syndrome have difficulty communicating their emotional state, and may move from anxiety to panic or tantrum without giving the usual warning signs that other children might provide. Thus, the child may be perceived as out of control, belligerent, hyperactive, or disobedient. It's important that families and teachers recognize the difference between children who "act out" for more typical reasons, and children who lose control because their anxieties have reached critical mass and produced a meltdown.

It's important to keep in mind that children with Asperger Syndrome, like all children, are individuals. Like all children, their personalities vary. Some may be quiet and prefer playing alone; others are more outgoing and intrusive. What they have in common are the underlying social difficulties that define this condition.

Asperger Syndrome and Autism

Because these social and emotional deficits are similar to those experienced by children with autism, Asperger Syndrome is part of what's called the "autism spectrum" of disabilities. Some use the term "high-functioning autism" to refer to this disorder, although experts are still studying and debating the precise relationship between Asperger Syndrome and higher-functioning autism. While the debate continues, it is probably most accurate to say that the conditions, if not indeed the same, do overlap. People with a diagnosis of higher-functioning autism have many of the same difficulties as those with Asperger Syndrome, and many of the ways of helping them cope with these difficulties are the same.

Despite the relationship between autism and Asperger Syndrome, the two disorders are strikingly different in impact on a child's life. The child with classic autism may also have mental retardation, or may have no language at all. Asperger Syndrome is often marked by average to superior intelligence and often precocious—if unusual—use of language. In addition, some children with autism seem to actively reject social contact. While some children with Asperger Syndrome are content by themselves, many would like very much to make friends.

Children with Asperger Syndrome often have an "adult" way of conversing that focuses on their fascination (or obsession) with a narrow subject. Such a child memorizes a vast fund of information and terminology about subway trains, butterflies, or black holes, and then dispenses this knowledge in situations where it may not always be appreciated.

Some children with Asperger Syndrome also meet the criteria of a condition called Nonverbal Learning Disability (NLD), which also is distinguished by difficulties in relating to others, using social language appropriately, and coping with the complexities of friendship and school activities. Children with NLD may have the same difficulty reading between the lines as children with Asperger Syndrome, but they generally do not have the fixated interests that so often identify Asperger Syndrome.

An important key to understanding Asperger Syndrome is the concept of "mindblindness" (described by Simon Baron-Cohen, in his book of the same name). It means an inability to put oneself in the place of another and to see things from another person's perspective. In recent years we have learned a great deal about the subtle yet essential skills involved in acquiring what is called "theory of mind." This capacity develops in children during the late preschool years, and enables them to perceive reality from another's perspective. This ability enables the child to feel empathy, to identify with another's feelings and point of view, and to understand that others don't know everything the child knows. It also makes it possible for the child to understand pretense, sarcasm, deceit, and certain kinds of humor.

We can think of Asperger Syndrome as a form of mental colorblindness. A person who is colorblind may have nearly normal vision and be able to cope quite well, except in certain situations when color identification is essential. In those situations, people usually compensate in some way and manage well—by memorizing the relative position of the traffic lights on the post, for example. Like the colorblind person, people with Asperger Syndrome can learn to compensate, can learn rules and techniques for getting on in the world.

Children with Asperger Syndrome may never develop a true theory of mind, or they may develop it slowly and with difficulty. In the meantime, they often possess a certain innocence, a lack of guile that can put them at greater risk of being misunderstood or victimized by others. Yet that same quality, along with honesty and a sense of fair play, can make them particularly endearing.

Many of the individual traits typical of Asperger Syndrome are found in typical children as well. Typical three-year-olds, for example, often display physical awkwardness or rote movements; bright four-year-olds may obsess about Thomas the Tank Engine or recite from memory dialog from favorite videos. Some bright five-year-olds, like Brendan, fall in love with maps and memorize the names of world capitals.

So it's essential to approach this subject with the understanding that not every child who exhibits some of these traits has the disorder. This book cannot offer a diagnosis for your child, although it will provide a road map for parents who are concerned about their child's development and are seeking information about a diagnosis.

Asperger Syndrome and "Genius"

Children with Asperger Syndrome are often intellectually precocious, and many grow up to have quite impressive skills in a particular area. Such "splinter" skills may include feats of calculation or memory, unusual abilities in music, or exceptional visual and spatial talents for engineering or architecture.

Unusual abilities in people who have other intellectual deficits are sometimes referred to as "savant" skills (in the case of people with mental retardation, the antiquated term "idiot savant" is sometimes used). But the term distracts us from our task of viewing the child with Asperger Syndrome as a whole, complex human being—one who, like everyone, has abilities that may cause difficulties, and also may cause great opportunity.

The same caution is appropriate when we discuss "genius" in connection with these unusual abilities. We usually associate that term with great accomplishment, whether or not the person has deficits. But often genius is accompanied by personal eccentricities: obsessive interests, social withdrawal, or odd ways of dressing and behaving. We picture Albert Einstein, shuffling around Princeton with his uncombed hair and his rumpled clothes, inventing brilliant mathematical formulas. This combination of brilliance and eccentricity has led to speculation that Einstein may have had Asperger Syndrome.

We'll never know for sure, of course. Whatever the connection may be between Asperger Syndrome and genius, we always need to keep foremost in our minds that unusual abilities (and uneven abilities) are part of the rich variety of the human family. As with everyone else, the success of children with Asperger Syndrome will depend on how they develop their abilities, and how successfully they are able to compensate for the difficult aspects of the condition. If your child can do these things, with your help, he may accomplish great things.

History

Our awareness of Asperger Syndrome has undergone a transformation since it was first described in 1944 by the Austrian physician Hans Asperger. Asperger's work was virtually ignored, especially in the United States, and the children who exhibited the unusual behavior he had observed were either written off as merely eccentric or peculiar, or they were lumped together with children with other diagnoses.

In 1981, British psychiatrist Lorna Wing published a paper on Asperger's work and her own observations that brought this syndrome to the attention of a wider audience. By the 1990s, the American Psychiatric Association recognized Asperger Syndrome as a diagnostic category, and in 1994 included it in the fourth edition of the *Diagnostic and Statistical Manual of Mental Disorders,* also known as DSM-IV.

The mid-1990s were a turning point for children and adults with Asperger Syndrome, and for their families. Finally, their condition had a recognized name and an official diagnosis. With this status came the hope for services and treatment. Since then, the number of children diagnosed with Asperger Syndrome has increased dramatically. Television programs and magazine articles have brought examples of real people with this disorder before the general public, and parents have become actively involved in increasing public awareness and lobbying for better educational opportunities and mental health services for their children.

Whether this increase reflects increased awareness or an increase in the actual prevalence of the condition is difficult to determine. The incidence of Asperger Syndrome in the U.S. population is impossible to state with precision; studies have indicated rates of anywhere from 1 in 10,000 to 7 in 1,000. The most recent reviews of the data have suggested a working figure of about 4 in 1,000. The condition is more prevalent in boys than in girls, perhaps as much as three times more so.

These estimates depend, in part, on how precise a definition is used. There is no simple test for Asperger Syndrome; it depends for the most part on careful observation of a child's behavior. There is a certain amount of "give" in the diagnostic criteria, so the accuracy of each diagnosis, and resulting population of people with the diagnosis, depends on the skill and experience of the team that makes the determination.

In some ways, we are fortunate that Asperger Syndrome is a recent diagnosis, at least in this country. Fifty years ago, the fields of psychology and medicine had a great deal to learn about genetics, neurology, and the science of behavior. Children with developmental disabilities, such as autism, were often treated as though they suffered from mental illness brought on by traumatic experiences or a lack of parental love. Such an approach not only failed to help the children, but brought untold suffering to their desperate parents as well.

We now know that Asperger Syndrome is the result of biological anomalies in the brain, which may have a genetic origin. The genetic explanation is somewhat complex, since most children do not have a parent with the condition. We'll discuss this dimension further in the following chapter.

Pervasive Developmental Disorders

Asperger Syndrome falls under the category of Pervasive Developmental Disorders, or PDDs, which includes autism. All five of the PDD diagnostic categories affect development in broad terms, and each varies significantly in the mix and severity of symptoms. Generally, Asperger Syndrome is less disabling than Autistic Disorder.

The five categories are as follows:

Autistic Disorder
Asperger Syndrome
Rett Syndrome
Childhood Disintegrative Disorder (CDD)
Pervasive Developmental Disorder: Not Otherwise Specified
    (PDD:NOS)

Each of the above conditions carries symptoms that can range from mild to severe. All are marked by characteristics in the four areas we have discussed: deficits in social abilities, impaired communication, odd behaviors or physical rituals, and unusual responses to stimuli. The differences involve the specific behaviors shown in each syndrome, and in the timing of the appearance of symptoms.

Autistic Disorder is characterized by severe deficits in social communication, to the point that the children may seem to live entirely in their own world. They may avoid eye contact and physical closeness. Some are unable to communicate at all; others may communicate only through gestures; others may use language but in unusual ways. They often engage in repetitive behaviors, from physical rocking and spinning, to head-banging or other self-stimulating behaviors, to obsessive focus on particular toys. Autism is more prevalent in boys, and is accompanied by mental retardation in about three quarters of individuals affected.

Rett Syndrome is a very rare genetic condition that affects primarily girls. It includes some of the motor and social disabilities found in autism and in Asperger Syndrome, but is marked by apparently normal early development, followed by a decline in skills. Girls with Rett Syndrome are sometimes incorrectly diagnosed with Autistic Disorder before age five, owing to the similarity of their problems.

Childhood Disintegrative Disorder (CDD) is very rare. It also is characterized by normal early development, often lasting several years, followed by a decline in development, in which language, motor skills, and self-care (such as toileting and dressing) regress to a degree consistent with a severe presentation of autism.

Finally, the category of Pervasive Developmental Disorder: Not Otherwise Specified (PDD:NOS) is reserved for individuals who show the three essential deficits of PDDs, but are difficult or impossible to classify. It allows children with a unique mixture of symptoms, who do not clearly fit under any of the other subcategories, to be classified under the PDD umbrella and receive a diagnosis that will enable us to better understand them, and assist them to get the help they need.

When parents of children with Asperger Syndrome learn that their child's condition is believed to be related to autism, they may react with fear and dread. Autism can be severely disabling. In addition, parents' only perception of autism may date from an era of ignorance, misunderstanding, and ineffective treatment options.

Yet a full understanding of the autistic spectrum is ultimately helpful, first because it provides a deeper understanding of the patterns of brain function that are involved across the spectrum, and second because it may reassure parents that Asperger Syndrome does tend to be among the less disabling of these disorders.

How Asperger Syndrome Affects Children and Families

Like any developmental disorder, Asperger Syndrome affects not only the child who has the condition, but the child's family and acquaintances as well. For parents, their child's disability not only can bring sorrow and worry, but can also be a blow to their self-esteem and confidence.

Asperger Syndrome can make it more likely that a child will behave not only oddly, but in ways that bring disapproval. When a child has a tantrum in public or appears to be socially withdrawn or inept, parents feel judged and scrutinized because of their child's behavior. One mother points with wry pride to the stunning perennial gardens in her yard. She planted them over one season when she had to stay home with her son, who refused to leave the house.

Sometimes parents avoid situations that bring discomfort, withdrawing from contact with relatives or acquaintances who seem unsympathetic. Parents of a typical child, for example, might have enjoyed taking that child to family gatherings or neighborhood picnics, where the adults relax as the children play nearby. But a younger child with Asperger Syndrome might change their social life entirely. The social gatherings become ordeals, as others criticize the child's outbursts or odd behavior.

They may have been active and appreciated volunteers at the older child's elementary school, but withdraw from those activities because the younger child's difficulties make them feel self-conscious. While this may be a reasonable approach in dealing with truly unsupportive people, this kind of withdrawal can lead to social and emotional isolation.

Siblings, also, must adjust to the brother or sister with Asperger Syndrome within the family, and adjust to the responses of others to that child. In addition, they may receive (or feel that they receive) less support from parents preoccupied with the needs of the disabled child.

When social difficulties continue into adolescence, the child with Asperger Syndrome may suffer from low self-esteem and depression. The child may experience anxiety and anger, both at home and in school situations. Of course, typical adolescents also experience self-doubt, feelings of inadequacy, and confusion about who they are and where they fit in. But teens with Asperger Syndrome have a much harder time building the peer supports that help typical adolescents through this stage of life. And when teenagers suffer, their families suffer along with them.

Raising a child with a disability puts a very real strain on families. The task can be more of a challenge when the disability is in some sense invisible; children with Asperger Syndrome are not visibly disabled, yet their behavior can cause tension within the family and make it difficult for parents to find baby sitters and other caregivers who might enable the parents to take a break.

And yet, families often report that their child's difficulties have brought them closer together. Married couples may find a renewed sense of mission and partnership as they share a child's daily setbacks and accomplishments. One mother had this to say:

"When your child begins to show signs of improvement, be they the tiniest steps, you want to sing for joy, but you'd feel like an idiot doing so. So I've shared these tiny yet momentous triumphs with my husband. *He* understood how incredible it was the first time our son got on the telephone and had an extended conversation with his uncle. *He* understood when we heard our son ask what a word meant. He got tears in his eyes when our son allowed a younger neighbor boy into his room and dragged out his box of Thomas trains for the child to play with. You see 'typical' kids do this stuff all the time, but other parents take it for granted. I don't believe my husband and I will ever take our son's achievements for granted."

And it's not just parents. Often, siblings and the extended family pull together for the child with Asperger Syndrome, sharing the burdens and celebrating the triumphs.

"There's nothing more wonderful," one parent told me, "than visiting extended family members who have not seen my son in a while—months or even years—and to witness their delighted shock at how he has improved."

Looking Ahead

Perhaps the most significant aspect of current studies of children with Asperger Syndrome is how hopeful the prognosis can be. With understanding and down-to-earth strategies for helping these children cope with their condition, their futures can be bright indeed.

As one parent puts it, "The diagnosis was certainly upsetting. But the encouraging news is that Andrew can learn to manage his disability. Asperger Syndrome shouldn't be thought of as a frightening label—facing it honestly is the first step in getting wonderful support and help, and learning to help your child."

As the parent of a child with Asperger Syndrome, you will find it helpful to remind yourself of these essential points: Yes, your child's condition is challenging. No, we don't have a "cure"—but then, such a drastic change would change who your child is. Asperger Syndrome has its place in the full range of human variation, and the world is a better place for this infinite variety of human traits and ways of thinking. You should allow yourself to take your full measure of delight in your child's uniqueness. We who work with children like yours are eager to find ways to help children be the best they can be, and to channel their strengths into creative places. When we discuss treating specific behaviors or problems, we are treating the difficult behaviors, not the child or the Asperger Syndrome.

As one mother puts it, "Asperger Syndrome is part of our diversity. I want Jessica to see it as part of the whole, wonderful, fantastic person she is. I want to teach her to cherish the many wonders of Asperger Syndrome, along with the need to meet the challenges it brings."

There are indeed challenges, but challenges are present in everyone's life. How we deal with them is the key to our futures, as one seventh-grade boy expressed so well: "We have difficulties like everyone else. But if someone works hard and makes the best of what they have, then it will not matter if they have a disability. They will be a success, Asperger Syndrome or not."

I would hope that you, as parents, relatives, or teachers of people with Asperger Syndrome—or as someone who has this condition yourself—will keep in mind several essential points. Despite some accounts in the media, Asperger Syndrome is not the same thing as precocity. Many bright, charming children with a fixation on their favorite subject are just that—bright, charming, focused children. Asperger Syndrome is quite different. It is a developmental disorder that brings many challenges, and those challenges must be addressed and taken seriously.

Asperger Syndrome is part and parcel of who the child is—as much as the color of his eyes. It is not something we separate out from him and "cure." Although it can be disabling, this condition brings with it many gifts and strengths. With wise and loving guidance, children who have Asperger Syndrome can become successful, independent adults—adults with difficulties, to be sure; adults with unique perspectives and talents, almost certainly.

2

The Trains Don't Always
Run on Time

What Is Going On Inside
My Child's Brain?

For Ethan, schedules have always been of paramount importance. He has always needed a timeline, and a plan to follow. Period. Ethan preferred being with those who understood this need for order best. That they were usually adults caused him no concern.

The world just didn't seem organized enough for this kindergartner. He became anxious if his books, videos, or favorite shirts weren't just where they were supposed to be. When things were changed, unpredictable, or happened unexpectedly, he would become very upset and have a tantrum. Understandably, trying to anticipate these situations and forestall their occurrence became a full-time job for his parents.

His mother tried to explain the importance of flexibility in life, but he didn't care. ("Straws and pipe cleaners were flexible," he commented. "How were people supposed to be like that?")

Everything changed one afternoon as Ethan and his family

were riding the train into New York. Ethan had loved trains for as long as he could remember, and given his exceptional memory, that was a long time! During the trip, he discovered the train schedule and realized, to his delight, that someone was creating a MetroNorth train schedule each and every day, and it was right there for him whenever he wanted it, on his computer.

Train schedules nearly became an obsession. The possibility of cancellations or delays became the focus of incessant question-asking and worry. His parents, like most commuters on MetroNorth, usually had no idea whatsoever as to the real causes of a delay or cancellation. They found it difficult to comfort Ethan.

Paradoxically, the thing that eventually helped tame the "Dragon of Orderliness" was another schedule. Ethan's parents decided to allow him to check the train schedule only twice each day. They wisely gave him some degree of control and choice in the matter, and issued him two "train schedule tickets" each morning, to be used at his discretion during the day. Once used, however, they were voided, just like a train ticket. Further, using the train schedule tickets implied a certain responsibility for behavior: no tantrums. This, they explained, was just like the conductor's expectation that passengers behave while riding the train.

This satisfied the "Dragon of Orderliness"—at least for a while. It was next sighted in the express checkout line (twelve items or less) of the local supermarket, when Ethan reached into the cart of a surprised shopper and removed items thirteen and fourteen.

Over the years, Ethan's parents have worked with him and his doctors to try to help him cope with his anxieties and his need to have everything remain soothingly the same. He is making progress. He and his parents understand that his behavior is probably biological in origin, but they still wonder where it comes from. In this chapter, we'll examine what is known about the biological foundation of Asperger Syndrome.

Not too long ago, a child with Asperger Syndrome would likely go undiagnosed and untreated. Or she might receive an incorrect diagnosis, and incorrect treatment. She might be labeled hyperactive, emotionally disturbed, obsessive-compulsive, or just plain spoiled. Her parents' questions about what caused her behavior would receive confusing or conflicting answers.

And, critically, no one would be able to explain what was going on in her brain, or in her environment, that contributed to her difficulties.

So often, subtle deficits in social functioning, or odd ways of relating to others or reacting to sensory stimuli, are attributed to upbringing. The child who has a tantrum when the ice cream parlor has run out of mint chocolate chip is viewed as spoiled. The child who removes extra items from a shopper's cart might be viewed with amused indulgence, but then again, he might not. The child who gives "sassy" answers is viewed as a brat. And that child's parents may receive a great deal of advice from friends, relatives, and strangers on the street.

"Everyone had a theory," one mother recalls. "I should be less controlling and give her more freedom. I should crack down and give her more limits. Whatever I was doing, whatever I'd just been told, was wrong."

It's certainly true that the behavior of parents can influence how well their child with Asperger Syndrome develops. But it's important to begin with what we know about the underlying biological origins of this disorder. This information helps parents in two ways. First, it should ease their suspicions that they may have caused their child's unusual behavior. And second, it helps parents identify effective ways of helping their child. The more we know about the activity within the brain of a child with Asperger Syndrome, the more effectively we can help her strengthen her weaknesses, compensate for her deficits, and play to her strengths.

What Research Is Revealing About Asperger Syndrome

From Lorna Wing's writings in the 1980s through 1994, when the American Psychiatric Association recognized Asperger Syndrome as a diagnostic category, we have made significant progress in our understanding of this condition. But the real impetus for this turnaround is the gradual evolution of our thinking about behavior from a strictly environmental model toward the more balanced model we use today, which acknowledges the interaction between environment and biology, between nurture and nature.

During the past fifty years, the way we view behavior has changed dramatically. At mid-century, most psychologists viewed environment and early experience as the essential determinants of behavior. Early trauma might contribute to anxieties, and cold or negligent parents could, it was believed, produce autism or schizophrenia in their offspring. Today, thanks to revolutions in biological research and brain imaging technology—and the resulting rethinking of nature versus nurture—we now understand the physical foundation of much of behavior, and the biological (and often genetic) origins of many behavioral disorders.

Currently, investigators are seeking a clearer genetic explanation of the Pervasive Developmental Disorders (PDDs). They are using marvelous technology to scrutinize the brain activity of living, thinking subjects to gain a clearer picture of where the crucial functions take place and how they differ from typical brains.

Someday, this research will yield valuable insights into the origins of Asperger Syndrome, and may help us modify some of its more difficult aspects. It will help us refine the interventions that we are using to help people with this disorder. But the chances are that the best approaches will continue to focus on those interventions—the teaching and practicing of social and conversational skills, and the modification of routines and environments.

Behavior—both positive and troublesome—surely results from the interaction between biology and environment. Your child's biological foundation and the environment you as a family provide interact to build her personality. With this understanding, we'll examine in this chapter what might be going on within the brain of Ethan and other children with Asperger Syndrome, and look at how the activity of his brain creates his behavioral tendencies. As parents, you will then be able to apply that understanding to your own child's behavior, and see how the techniques we will discuss later in this book mesh with—and compensate for—the particular deficits in brain function.

A Note About Alternative "Causes" of Autism Spectrum Disorders

As far as we know at this point, Asperger Syndrome is caused by anomalies in the brain that are present at birth. Its underlying cause is probably genetic, although other factors may contribute to how it is expressed, or to the severity of the disorder.

It should be noted that in recent years, other possible causes of autism spectrum disorders have been discussed in the scientific journals, the mainstream media, and even congressional hearings. Thus far, none of the alternative theories—from allergies to food additives to vitamin deficiencies—has been found to have a clear scientific basis.

One of the best known of these alternative theories is the speculation of a link between autistic disorders and childhood immunization. Research in England, and reports from parents in the United States and abroad, has claimed a link between the MMR (measles-mumps-rubella) vaccine and the development of autism. However, other research has failed to establish any link. Some observers point out that the theory gained credibility among some parents because the immunization schedule coincides with the ages at which symptoms of autistic disorders become apparent. In addition, the incidence of autism has increased over the same period of time that childhood immunization has become widespread. Experts believe the increased incidence of autistic disorders is not related to immunization rates, but rather to greater awareness among parents and professionals, and because of broader definitions of autism spectrum disorders, including Asperger Syndrome.

Social Learning in the "Typical" Brain

Human beings are by nature social animals, and as such, our brains are "hard-wired" from the earliest stages of development for social behavior. Newborn infants recognize their caregivers by smell and show preference for their mothers' scent; this behavior is not something they have to be taught. As their brains and experience blossom, they acquire the social abilities that will link them to those they depend on, and provide pleasure and reward for behavior that fosters attachment.

Thus, babies gurgle and smile at their parents; they soon smile and laugh, and later they offer toys to visitors and wave goodbye. As they venture outside the family, they learn to take turns, to follow certain rules, and to restrain some of their impulses in social settings. All these abilities come about through an interaction between their developing brains and learning opportunities provided by their environment.

Although we don't have a great deal of data on infant behavior in Asperger Syndrome, most parents report that their babies showed typical behavior. They displayed a social smile, engaged in reciprocal babbling, and developed "shared attention"—pointing to a truck, for example, and turning to the mother to include her in the experience. This is not the case in autism, in which many parents report unusual behavior from infancy, including avoidance of eye contact, lack of apparent interest in others, and delayed language acquisition.

If brain development is delayed, or in some way hampered, however, social learning in early childhood is much more difficult. Let's go back to the concept we discussed in chapter 1 called "theory of mind."

How We Learn to Think About Thinking

Theory of mind is not the kind of thing we spend our time thinking about—we just do it. We have a PIN for our bank account, which means only we can get money from an automatic teller machine, because other people don't have the same information we do. We smile and give a friendly greeting to someone we don't really wish to see, because we want to be kind; we know that the other person isn't reading our thoughts. We play poker, or bid at an auction, or engage in seduction, always with an awareness of the difference between our own state of mind and that of another.

This ability to make the distinction between our own thoughts and knowledge and the thoughts and knowledge of others is crucial. It allows us to lie and deceive, to be sure—but it also allows us to care about other people, to engage in irony, to appreciate humor, and to create imaginary images in art or drama. When it is impaired, we are less able to sympathize with others, or to anticipate the effect of our behavior or words on others.

Children are remarkably consistent in the age at which they acquire this ability. It occurs about the age of four in most children. Three-year-olds are easy to fool, and tend to think literally. Five-year-olds are much harder to deceive, and in fact can be deceitful themselves.

The classic experiment that demonstrates the acquisition of this ability, called the Sally-Anne Experiment, was developed by Heinz Wimmer and Josef Perner and uses two dolls, one who has a basket, and the other a box. The experimenter shows children Sally, with her basket, and Anne, with her box, and has Sally put a marble in her basket. Sally then departs, and Anne takes the marble and hides it in her own container. Then Sally returns, and the experimenter asks the crucial question: Where will Sally look for her marble?

Three-year-old children respond that Sally will look in the box. That's where the marble is, after all; they *saw* Anne put it there. They assume Sally knows it as well.

Four-year-olds, however, are more shrewd. They know that although they saw Anne move the marble, Sally did not, and thus does not share their knowledge.

The development of this understanding marks a significant step in a child's journey toward maturity. The four-year-old has, in a sense, tasted the fruit of the Tree of Knowledge and understands much of the complexity of the world. The child who has not developed the ability to consider the state of mind of another is still living in a state of innocence that makes it difficult to navigate the complexities of the social world.

Recently, researchers have used brain imaging technology to attempt to locate the region of the brain where this kind of thinking occurs. Positron emission tomography (PET) and functional magnetic resonance imaging (fMRI) can illuminate activity in specified regions of the brain; researchers can ask the subject to answer a question or perform a task and observe what regions this particular task activates.

Thus, research has revealed that subjects with Asperger Syndrome rely on different regions than do typical subjects when asked to imagine another's state of mind. The same is true when subjects are asked to identify faces and to evaluate facial expressions.

Clearly, the brain's ability not only to perceive the state of mind of others, but to recognize and evaluate the many hints that other people offer about their state of mind, is diminished in people with Asperger Syndrome.

As we will see in the discussion below, other brain regions and other functions contribute to the particular difficulties of Asperger Syndrome, but this theory of mind aspect appears to be of particular importance.

Brain Structure and Pervasive Developmental Disorders

Although the body of research into Asperger Syndrome and its relationship to brain structure and function is small, it is growing. More research has been conducted on patients with autism, and much of that data can be applied to Asperger Syndrome as well, since the deficits are similar.

The Cerebellum

It has been known for some time that people with autism tend to have abnormalities in the structure and function of the cerebellum, the primitive region in the back of the brain that regulates balance and spatial perception. Researcher Eric Courchesne reported that a majority of his patients with autism had cerebellums that are substantially smaller than in typical people. This abnormality may account for some of the motor deficits and awkwardness found in patients with PDDs, including Asperger Syndrome.

But its impact may go beyond the scope of physical coordination. Stroke patients with damage to the cerebellum, for example, may have the physical strength and ability to walk, but they may have great difficulty on stairs, or may have to look at their feet as they walk, because they have lost the sense of their body's position in space.

Courchesne conducted studies comparing the performance of people with damaged cerebellums and people with autism. In both, the ability to switch attention from one stimulus to another is impaired, meaning that these subjects must focus intently on each stimulus as it comes into view before being able to move on to another.

This inability to switch one's attention smoothly from one stimulus to another, Courchesne suggests, contributes to the difficulty that autistic persons have comprehending a complex whole. It may contribute to their tendency to perceive the world as a series of unrelated pieces, rather than as an integrated whole. Surely this deficit would contribute to difficulty "reading" facial expressions, for example. It might also contribute to the difficulty people with Asperger Syndrome have in smoothly processing social communication on many levels: what other people are saying, the emotional meaning behind their words, and their body language.

The Limbic System

The more primitive regions of the brain, including the cerebellum, control the most basic functions, such as balance, respiration, and involuntary responses. Situated between those primitive structures and the higher-function region of the cerebral cortex is a network of structures called the limbic system, where emotions are generated and directed. The limbic system is not where subtle, sophisticated sensibilities exist—that is the realm of the cortex. The limbic system handles fear, lust, joy, anger, and all those basic emotions that draw us toward positive experiences and help us escape unpleasant or dangerous ones.

Recent research has pointed to a particular structure in the limbic system that may be at the heart of the social and emotional difficulties associated with Asperger Syndrome. This structure—actually two small almond-shaped structures—is called the amygdala.

The amygdala is situated in a sort of command central within the brain, with links to all the senses and to the more analytical areas of the cortex. Its function is to receive sensory input, quickly determine its emotional content, and send the appropriate message both to the cortex, for thoughtful sorting, and to the hypothalamus, a limbic structure that triggers hormone responses.

Thus, a snarling dog causes visual and auditory signals to be received and sent to the amygdala, which attaches a "fear" or "danger" marker on the experience. It signals the hypothalamus to trigger the release of cortisone (adrenaline), and the cortex to think about dogs and how to escape from dangerous ones.

Research by Yale psychologist Robert T. Schultz and others suggests that abnormalities in the amygdala explain at least part of the symptoms of Asperger Syndrome. Because this structure is so richly connected to the parts of the cortex that govern social and emotional functioning, abnormalities can hinder these connections and result in behavioral deficits. Damage to the amygdala can hinder the brain's ability to assign emotional meaning to situations, and that inability can, in turn, hinder emotional learning—both essential in reading social situations and determining how to respond in them.

The Cerebral Cortex

The cortex—the fissured "gray matter" of our image of the brain—is where higher functions such as reasoning and planning occur. The cortex is highly differentiated, with different regions handling different functions, and researchers have been able to learn a great deal recently about this differentiation by tracing brain activity, as mentioned above, and by detecting physical abnormalities in brain structures.

But most of our intellectual functions are not limited to one isolated organ or region. Most require coordination among several regions. Language, for example, requires both Broca's area (which copes with vocabulary) and Wernicke's region (which handles grammar). And the left hemisphere of the brain is the locale of the structure of language, while the right hemisphere deals with its emotional content.

Similarly, other regions appear to be activated when we experience emotions, attempt to read facial expressions, and make social judgments. Deficits in the temporal lobes, for example, can lead to poor recognition of facial expressions, and difficulty in detecting the emotional states that facial expressions suggest (the distinction between a look of consternation and a look of anger, for example).

Particular regions appear to be associated with "theory of mind," as we discussed previously in this chapter. Prefrontal cortex deficits appear related to difficulties with assigning mental states to others—essential in predicting how another person might respond to a situation.

All this would suggest that many of the difficulties experienced by people with Asperger Syndrome are likely to be traceable to abnormalities in structure or function of particular regions of the brain.

Executive Function

As we have seen, the details of the brain can be functioning properly, and yet more complex aspects of thinking can be impaired. We are learning more about the subtle aspects of brain function that tend to go unnoticed when they are working well, but which can cause great difficulties when they aren't.

One example of this is what we call "executive function." This is the term we use for those critical reasoning and judgment skills that permit interpretation of events, process feedback, and foster flexibility and divergent thinking. It makes divergent thinking—thinking "outside the box"—possible. More important, executive function is the kind of thinking that tells us when we *ought* to think outside the box. Without it, or when it is impaired, people have difficulty navigating life's ups and downs, and readjusting their behavior and thinking when things aren't working.

Executive function is a high-level cortical ability, and while it's a form of intelligence, it takes place quite separately from the kind of cognitive activity that we think of as intelligence. People with impaired executive function may achieve very high IQ scores, but have great difficulty planning, organizing their time and their surroundings, and managing their lives.

For those of us with typical brains, it's sometimes difficult to imagine some of the challenges experienced by people with Asperger Syndrome. Most of us have no difficulty recognizing faces, picking up nonverbal cues or body language, or learning the basics of etiquette. But executive function deficits are things we can all imagine, because we all have failures in this area from time to time.

When we forget where we put our glasses or car keys, when we simply can't get around to calculating our taxes, when we have attacks of disorganization, or when we struggle with decisions about our next career move, we are experiencing perfectly normal shortcomings in this important function. What's different about people with Asperger Syndrome is that these shortfalls occur more often and are much more difficult to overcome.

A child with Asperger Syndrome, asked to clear the dinner table, may comply by picking up one knife, carrying it to the kitchen, and then returning for another. When asked to clean her bedroom, she may well become overwhelmed. What seems like a simple task actually embodies a whole array of small, but crucial decisions: Shall I keep this or throw it away? If I keep it, where should I put it? Shall I start by making the bed, or picking things up off the floor, or cleaning my desk, or emptying my closet?

An adult with Asperger Syndrome may have the same difficulty organizing her home or apartment, keeping important records, planning a job search, or arranging a vacation. Even such basic tasks as getting up in the morning to go to work involve executive function: the desire to turn off the alarm clock and roll over can easily override the cerebral messages warning us of dire consequences if we do.

Genetics

Information about the human genetic structure has grown enormously in the past few years, with the recent mapping of the human genome. That map, however, is a starting point; it does not tell us all we will eventually know about the link between particular behaviors and disorders and particular genes.

Although it is unlikely we'll find a specific "Asperger Syndrome gene" in the near future, it is likely that within the next decade a much clearer picture of the genetic underpinning of Asperger Syndrome will emerge.

There is considerable evidence of a family history in Asperger Syndrome, although it is not evident in all cases. What is more likely is that a tendency toward the spectrum of PDDs runs in some families, with the particular diagnosis and severity depending on as yet unknown factors.

Thus, many parents are able to describe a relative with unusual symptoms or behaviors—someone who was a "loner," "eccentric," or just socially awkward. Their observations are supported by research by Susan Folstein, a physician at Tufts University, into what is described as the "broader autism phenotype"—the presence of one or more traits that, in isolation, do not constitute a disability, but which are combined in individuals diagnosed with autism spectrum disorders.

For example, a parent may be described in one or more of the following ways: rigid, resistant to change, having a preference for solitary activities, having some oddities in conversation, or being disorganized, absent-minded, or having other executive function difficulties.

An individual with any one of these traits certainly would not be described as having a developmental disorder; indeed, many such people live successful and fulfilling lives. Estimates are that about 4 percent of the population possesses this phenotype. But in families in which a child has Asperger Syndrome, about 25 percent of the parents studied exhibit the broader autism phenotype, suggesting that it is inherited, and that the disorders themselves emerge depending on subtle genetic combinations.

Hypersensitivity

We all vary greatly in terms of our innate sensitivity to sensory stimuli. Some of us can sleep undisturbed through a mighty racket while others are awakened by the slightest sound. Some of us are tone-deaf, while others have exquisitely sensitive hearing (or sense of smell or taste). These are normal variations in the way our brains function.

Children with Asperger Syndrome often have acute senses. Some appear to possess normal senses but respond to them with more intensity. As we noted in chapter 1, they may smell odors undetectable to others. Or they may hear noises in the same way as most people, but respond to them with great distress or panic. One adult with Asperger Syndrome who is a brilliant musician and composer recalls that as a child, she would burst into tears when the piano was even slightly out of tune.

Although we are not sure precisely why these experiences are common, we suspect that they relate not so much to the senses themselves as they do to the limbic system and its way of processing incoming information.

When sensory stimuli are difficult to process, they can feel less like incoming information, and more like incoming artillery. Most of us would do whatever we could to escape an attack; children with unusual sensitivity react to being overwhelmed in ways that may appear odd to people with typical senses.

Thus, the child with Asperger Syndrome panics at the sound of a vacuum cleaner, refuses to eat foods that most children like, refuses to wear clothing that feels "scratchy," or falls apart emotionally at a lively birthday party. Although the senses themselves may be particularly intense, it is usually the way in which the limbic system treats these stimuli, and links them with distress, that causes such difficulty in children with Asperger Syndrome.

What Our Understanding of the Brain Tells Us

The more we understand how the brain functions, the more we are able to consider how a child with Asperger Syndrome views the world, and how much of the behavior that seems to be causing her trouble is actually the result of her effort to compensate for deficits. A child in a stressful situation, for example, may sense that she needs to gather her strength, and thus reaches for the area in which she is confident, no matter how inappropriate.

Children who feel overwhelmed by change in routine, or by new and confusing situations, may seek comfort and solace in physical behavior that calms them, such as rocking, or fidgeting, even though by so doing they draw attention to themselves.

British researcher Uta Frith has conducted extensive studies on how children with autistic spectrum disorders view the world. She believes that what is lacking in their way of thinking is "central coherence"—that cohesive force that is so strong in typical brains that we ordinarily are unaware of it.

For example, children with a weaker cohesive force tend to view fragments of their environment, rather than take in an organized whole. In what's called an "embedded figure test," they will do particularly well at picking out an image that is hidden, or embedded, in a larger figure. They are able to easily override this cohesive sense that presses most of us to look at an image as a whole.

Similarly, Frith's subjects with autism were able to memorize strings of nonsense words quite well; they performed about the same when asked to memorize meaningful words in a sentence. Typical children had difficulty remembering the nonsense words, but did much better with strings of words that "made sense."

Indeed, those of us with typical brains have great difficulty overriding this compulsion to "make sense" of things. That's why we have trouble picking out a picture of a monkey that is embedded within a larger picture of a forest. We enjoy optical illusions, in which our brains fool our eyes by imposing sense on an ambiguous image.

So much that is difficult for children with Asperger Syndrome can be explained in terms of this cohesion model; conversation and social conventions involve not so much small, mathematically accurate behaviors or statements, but overall sensing of the situation, of the mind states of others, of what's best in a particular situation.

That trouble with context may contribute to the sometimes startling literalism displayed by some children with Asperger Syndrome. David was often confused by simple statements such as "Take a chair" or "Hold the door." When his teacher said, "Can you show me your homework?" David would say, "Yes," without showing her anything, thinking he had answered the question accurately. He had indicated his ability to show his homework, but failed to interpret her words correctly. The teacher's comments on his report card described him as "belligerent" and "fresh."

Despite his above-average verbal skills, David's use and understanding of language remain highly literal. He is unable to grasp the more subtle uses of language, such as idiomatic expressions, irony, and certain kinds of humor.

. . .

We can see, then, how a child with Asperger Syndrome might focus on a narrow interest, rather than the subject's broader context—an obsessive interest in the uniforms of professional basketball teams, for example, with no interest whatever in the actual games.

We can see how social cues and facial expressions might be missed or misinterpreted by a child whose interest was hijacked by a fascinating image—the other person's necktie, for example, or earrings, or cologne.

We can see how upsetting change might be when every new situation threatens to overwhelm the child's ability to make sense of all the pieces. Elena, who is eleven, arises every morning at 5:30, gets the newspaper, and reads the comics before getting ready for school. A benign routine—until the day comes that the newspaper isn't delivered on time. For Elena, this alteration in her routine is not a minor disappointment, but a devastating blow to her equilibrium. It isn't possible for Elena to put the newspaper routine into perspective, because perspective and proportion are the areas she has trouble with. Her routines are lifelines, and she depends on them to get through her day.

When senses and information come in as fragments, when the cohesion function is impaired and the tendency to assign meaning to information is weakened, then experience is by definition unexpected, unpredictable, surprising, startling. In a sense, you can never let your guard down; you never know what's going to pop out from behind a door. In his book, *Shadow Syndromes,* psychiatrist John Ratey describes a man who became anxious about the very idea of doorways. His anxiety derived from the fact that a doorway often becomes occupied by a person—a person who arrives through the doorway and changes everything, demanding responses, altering the routine.

One can understand the appeal, or sense of comfort, that a child might find in repetitive behaviors, or information gathering, in a controlled setting. What's crucial about the narrow interests typical of Asperger Syndrome (maps, trains, ZIP codes, etc.) is their isolation. Any of these interests could be extended to a broader, coherent subject, but in Asperger Syndrome usually remain disconnected, although, as we'll discuss in later chapters, the intense interests of young children can often be expanded into a productive interest or career.

When we understand what is going on in the mind of a child with Asperger Syndrome, what underlies the need for routine, the difficulty making sense of social conventions, and the appeal of a particular comforting interest or hobby, then we are more able to direct that child toward behavior that not only will ease her mind, but will help her cope with school, work, friendships, and life.

The earlier we can identify what is not typical about the child with Asperger Syndrome, the more able we are to intervene in ways that allow the most opportunity for development. Schultz and others suggest that the structural deficits in the brains of people with Asperger Syndrome may not be enough, on their own, to explain the condition. What those deficits may do is create missed opportunities for social learning in the child. Thus, an impaired ability to share an emotional experience with a parent at one year of age, or, at age four, to theorize about what another person is thinking, means that the learning built on those experiences may be lost. The same might be true for the inability to process several stimuli at the same time, to sort out important stimuli from background noise, and other skills that form the foundation of intellectual and social development.

Some of that learning we can re-create. We can compensate to some degree for the deficits we find in the brain. Thus, we can offer techniques that help your child learn more of what she needs to know, at a more appropriate age, so that while she retains the remarkable brain structure that nature gave her, she can develop skills that will help her cope with the world and make the most of her gifts.

3

He's Ready for His World, But I'm Not

Getting, and Coping with, a Diagnosis

The following is the reaction of a patient's mother to her son's diagnosis.

"Your son has Asperger Syndrome." I never anticipated that hearing those words out loud would be so difficult for me.

After all, I have been going to a support group for kids with sensory integration issues, PDD:NOS, and high-functioning autism, for several months. Ethan definitely has sensory issues and motor planning problems, but any idea of autism was something I did not want to hear.

There was comfort in not having a diagnosis, a hope, and a denial that whatever my gut said, however much he seemed to "fit" on the "spectrum," I would be proven wrong by medical science. "My son has Asperger Syndrome." I run away from those words, shy away, flee. It startles me when I hear my husband say it out loud to a friend. I want to gather my son in my arms, and run to a safe place, and shut out the world.

I know so little about it. I have resisted knowing. I buy books and don't read them. I say to my husband, "You please read the books and be in charge of knowing what it's all about, what Ethan needs." Right now, I do not want to know. I do not want to answer any questions people may have. I panic when my husband's sister calls and asks me, "Does he really have autism? Does he flap his hands?" My father-in-law is devastated, remorseful, and guilty. "Is it my genes?" he wants to know.

I stumble at the phrase "Asperger Syndrome." Visions of the movie *Rain Man* fill me with dread. What will be Ethan's place in the world? How can we help him, guide him through life? It is all so overwhelming. Even though I went into the doctor's office with some knowledge, hearing what she had to say broke me wide open. I so wanted to hear, "Ethan is fine, just delayed, can be fixed quickly with a prescription." I still do not want to hear those words regarding my son. I do not want to share this information with anyone, not family, friends, or school. I want to keep it buried within our immediate family, keep it quiet, secret, only for us. It feels too real, too final. I want to protect my son, wrap him in a shield of blankets, and hold him close.

Yet, Ethan himself wants to be independent.

We say goodbye at the school door each morning after our walk there. He puts his arm out to push at me. "Don't come in, Mom," he commands.

He is ready, even eager, for his world.

I am not.

An accurate diagnosis of Asperger Syndrome is likely to be a turning point for your family. It may bring an end to the fog of confusion that you've felt about your child's problems. It means letting go of a certain hope you may have been clinging to—hope that your child will grow out of his problems, or that there is an easy cure, and all will be well tomorrow.

Like this mother, you may find that learning the truth is agonizing. It calls up a whole range of emotions, about many facets of your life. Your relationship with your own parents, your spouse or partner, and your other children will be reexamined in the light of this new knowledge: Why me? Do I have some of these traits? Was my own father's withdrawn behavior attributable to Asperger Syndrome?

And yet with this knowledge comes power. Many families have told me that when they finally learned what their child had, they felt a sense of great relief.

In this chapter we will discuss the journey toward an accurate and useful diagnosis, and then come back to the feelings this knowledge will bring you. The diagnosis itself is only the beginning. How you handle the news, and how you harness your knowledge to help your child, are the real challenges. This is not to minimize the struggle many families have arriving at that diagnosis in the first place. In fact, until recently, this disorder was so little known that misdiagnosis (or no diagnosis at all) was the norm. "Up until very recently, everybody was misdiagnosed," said one parent who heads a regional support group for families of children with Asperger Syndrome. "All adults were misdiagnosed. Many were labeled autistic and unsalvageable."

Much of the confusion, of course, stems from the fact that there was no recognized diagnostic category for Asperger Syndrome until 1994 (although some experts used the term and offered appropriate treatments before that). But even in recent years, many parents of children with Asperger Syndrome have had great difficulty getting anyone to evaluate their child thoroughly and accurately. They report a seemingly endless search for someone, anyone, who will understand their child, who will unlock the secret. They devote years and fortunes to therapy with psychologists who may miss the point entirely. One psychologist told a parent simply, "His problem is, he's too bright."

Many have felt the need to become lay experts on their own, or pursue advanced degrees, the better to understand and support their child.

Even now, diagnosis of Asperger Syndrome is a complex process. The evaluation itself is not a simple task; unlike some conditions that can be detected with a simple test, Asperger Syndrome is diagnosed through careful observation of symptoms that are, by their nature, subtle. And it requires an unhurried observation of the child.

What seem like precocious verbal skills in a child may be just that: precocious skills in an otherwise typical child. Usually it's the social deficits that draw parents' attention, and lead to an evaluation. Yet even these social deficits need to be carefully distinguished from social awkwardness that many children exhibit, or from other disorders that may explain them.

Let's look at two second graders, both bright, but both also somewhat shy and introverted.

Tommy learned to read easily before kindergarten, is very good with computers, and has recently become an expert chess player. The same is true of Jed. Tommy gets along well with two or three kids who also like chess or computers. Here, Jed has a harder time. When he plays chess, he always needs to have the white pieces. If he can't, he raises his voice and insists loudly. When his best friend no longer liked playing chess, Jed no longer wanted to do things with him. Tommy's friends know he is a good sport when they want to play something else besides chess or computer games, because he usually goes along with the group. Not Jed. It's his way or no way, as the other kids liked to say; his rules or nothing. The other children put up with it sometimes, but not for long.

Tommy is also a good friend when something isn't quite right with a classmate. He makes sure his friends aren't left out of a group, and he often goes to play with them if they're alone at recess. Jed approaches things differently. He has a hard time understanding why other kids get so upset about things. Sometimes he just tells them to "Stop it!" and walks away.

The teacher thinks Tommy is a bit too quiet for his own good. Sometimes, even when he knows the answer to a question in class, he won't raise his hand. He answers cheerfully if called upon, however. If he gives the wrong answer, he just takes it in stride.

Not so for Jed. He raises his hand whether he knows the correct answer or not, and wants to be called on each time. Sometimes he will just say whatever is on his mind, like what he saw on Scooby-Doo the day before. If his teacher tries to redirect him, he resists and keeps bringing up the same topic. If she corrects him, things sometimes get worse. When he's upset, Jed starts talking about his lists: lists of PG movies he wants to see, the actors in those movies, lists of animals he has studied, lists of iguanas and where they live. He isn't easy to distract, and when he *really* gets upset about being corrected, he paces back and forth while shaking his hands at his sides. When these things happen, the kids in his class, even Tommy, get a little nervous and wonder what is wrong with him.

Tommy is a bright, somewhat introverted child who has intense interests. Jed shares these qualities, but also has traits that suggest Asperger Syndrome: his difficulty adjusting his behavior to signals given by others, his trouble seeing things from another point of view, the anxiety he exhibits at the smallest change in routine.

Asperger Syndrome affects children differently, and sometimes behavior associated with it can appear subtle at first glance. By comparing a child's behavior to the actions of other children his age, however, it is often possible to see the unusual variations that are excessively rigid, naive, one-sided, or egocentric despite obvious academic strengths.

Early Indications of Asperger Syndrome

The parents of Ethan (whom we also met in chapter 2) tell the story of the moment when they first realized something was unique about their son. One day, when he was nearing his second birthday, he was riding in the back seat of the car when the Grateful Dead came on the car radio.

"By the second chorus," his parents recall, "we could hear from the back, as if from a tinny, treble stereo speaker, a tiny voice chirping with the band:

> *Driving that train*
> *High on cocaine . . .*

"We were astonished, amused, and a little concerned that our toddler was already parroting, if not comprehending, the vocabulary of drugs. It wasn't until later that we realized the true source of his interest in the song was its mention of trains."

Often, the first sign parents get that there may be something unusual about their child is an unusual facility with language (singing along with Jerry Garcia before age two, for example), or an intense interest in a particular subject that is more persistent than that of most small children.

However, in many cases, parents notice nothing unusual at all about their child's early development, and this is a major point of difference between Asperger Syndrome and autism.

In classic autism, children show unusual behavior quite early. As infants, they may be irritable, and may stiffen and resist when picked up by their parents. They may not develop a social smile, and refuse to make eye contact as toddlers. They may not speak at all. These children usually get evaluated at an early age.

Because Asperger Syndrome does not usually appear in infancy, often the first evidence that a child is in any way unusual is in his precocity. He reads stop signs at age two. At the breakfast table, he nibbles his toast into a map of Minnesota.

As he grows older, the parents may perceive the child's intense interest in maps and geography as dedication; a seriousness of purpose that explains his preference for playing alone, or only in parallel play—the visiting child wants to play "pretend," but the child with Asperger Syndrome will cooperate only as long as he can manipulate his maps and globes.

The Advantages and Disadvantages of Early Diagnosis

Because deficits are usually observed in social and peer settings, Asperger Syndrome may not be suspected before the beginning of school. Even then, an actual diagnosis may take time.

It's not uncommon for young children to receive an initial diagnosis of PDD:NOS (Pervasive Developmental Disability: Not Otherwise Specified), which may later be refined more precisely as Asperger Syndrome. While parents who suspect their child has Asperger Syndrome may dispute this diagnosis, it is often an appropriate clinical judgment. It allows the child to receive support in school and elsewhere, and allows time for the final diagnosis to be made when the social difficulties and eccentric, intense interests of later childhood emerge. A diagnosis within the PDD spectrum allows the appropriate interventions to be undertaken early, even though the specific diagnosis may have to wait until the child grows older and exhibits symptoms of Asperger Syndrome more clearly.

Conversely, a premature diagnosis of Asperger Syndrome in a young child who has another condition may not only mislead parents, but provide erroneous information to educators.

Some of the substantial increase in diagnosis of Asperger Syndrome over the past five years may be due not only to better diagnostic procedures but to inaccurate but well-meaning clinicians who believe the diagnosis to be more acceptable than autism, or more precise than PDD:NOS.

That said, there are distinct advantages to being aware of your child's difficulties early. As we said in the first chapter, some of the deficits, although organic in origin, may be magnified by the lessened opportunities for social learning that the brain abnormalities cause. Thus, if you observe that your four-year-old is having trouble making friends, or initiating social conversations, you might pursue a diagnosis.

The Perils of Misdiagnosis

Peter, a nine-year-old who is large for his age, seemed out of control in the classroom. He seemed to provoke the other students with inappropriate comments. He had outbursts of anger when he became upset.

He was diagnosed as having Oppositional Defiant Disorder, in which a child is consistently defiant and disobedient. He was placed in a classroom with other children whose behavioral difficulties stemmed from emotional problems.

Naturally, Peter's symptoms grew worse. The other kids scared him. His anxiety increased. And his social skills not only didn't improve, they deteriorated. He alternated between copying the worst behavior of the other children and being teased and victimized by them. Peter actually had Asperger Syndrome, and the placement of a child with a social language disorder in a classroom of children who are emotionally disabled was devastating.

Peter did eventually have an appropriate evaluation and was placed in a better setting, but misdiagnosis such as he experienced is not unusual. Of course, false identification is a two-way street; sometimes children are identified as having Asperger Syndrome when in fact they have another disorder entirely. This is a risk when any condition is new; unseasoned but enthusiastic practitioners may see it when it's not really there.

But a greater concern is when Asperger Syndrome is diagnosed as something else. Not only does misdiagnosis cause lost opportunities for the kinds of interventions that will help, it also exposes children to treatments and placements that are entirely inappropriate, as they were for Peter.

In addition to a diagnosis of emotional disturbance, children with Asperger Syndrome may receive one of the following labels.

· *Attention Deficit Disorder (ADD) or Attention Deficit Hyperactivity Disorder (ADHD).* This is one condition that may have suffered from overdiagnosis in recent years. Some children who were gathered under the label of ADD have since been more correctly identified as having Asperger Syndrome. It's an understandable mistake, since children with Asperger Syndrome may show many of the symptoms of restlessness, inattention, and poor academic focus common in ADD. However, the error can lead to inappropriate use of medication.

· *Mental retardation.* Although most children with Asperger Syndrome test within the normal range on standard IQ tests (and often above the normal range), their scores are uneven, showing deficits in select verbal and nonverbal areas. Their difficulties with pragmatic language also can be misinterpreted as evidence of retardation. Clearly, programs for children with mental retardation would be inappropriate for children with Asperger Syndrome, who often learn and retain information quickly. Their deficits are in unraveling the complexities of social interaction. A placement with children who have mental retardation would frustrate a child with Asperger Syndrome, and fail to address his need for practice in negotiating the social world of typical children.

· *Nonverbal Learning Disability (NLD).* Although Asperger Syndrome and NLD are considered distinct categories, in most cases interventions are similar and an error in diagnosis early on is not likely to be damaging. Children with NLD have many of the same social and pragmatic language difficulties, but are less likely to exhibit the intense, single-minded focus that children with Asperger Syndrome do.

· *Autism.* As we've said, there is some overlap in the behavior and needs of people with Asperger Syndrome and high-functioning autism. Whether they are indeed the same disorder remains a topic of vigorous discussion in the research community, but the practical interventions are fairly similar. What causes difficulty is when a diagnosis of autism steers professionals toward interventions that are more appropriate for children with the classic, severe form. And such a diagnosis might cause parents to adopt inaccurate expectations of their child's future capabilities.

· *PDD:NOS.* Of all the likely incorrect diagnoses, this is the least problematical. Often, it's appropriate for young children who may not clearly exhibit all the hallmarks of Asperger Syndrome. Interventions that you might use for a child with PDD:NOS are likely to be the same ones you'd use if the child had a label of Asperger Syndrome early on.

·   *Schizophrenia.* As we described earlier, some children with highly sensitive hearing or other senses can appear to be suffering from delusions or hallucinations to those with typical senses. A diagnosis of schizophrenia would lead to entirely inappropriate interventions, and could be particularly dangerous because management of schizophrenia usually involves the use of powerful drugs. Such a misdiagnosis is rare, however, because schizophrenia is rare in children under age fifteen, and most professionals would be highly wary of such a diagnosis.

In addition, diagnoses such as Obsessive-Compulsive Disorder, Oppositional Defiant Disorder, and Anxiety Disorder (or a combination of these) may be given.

Asperger Syndrome is a chronic condition. You, as parents, will need to monitor its course and development. Your child's initial diagnosis, whether correct or not, is just the beginning of a lifelong process of assessing your child's needs and providing the appropriate interventions.

Initiating the Evaluation

Usually the first person to realize that a child needs to be evaluated for Asperger Syndrome is the parent. You may have noticed that your preschooler shows little interest in peers, or that your kindergarten child seems abnormally upset by changes in routine or by noisy environments that most children love. You may have heard about Asperger Syndrome or autism and approached your pediatrician with your concerns.

Frequently, parents do not observe their young child in the intense social setting of kindergarten or elementary school. Often an observant teacher who knows what to expect of typical children picks up unusual behavior in the classroom.

Sometimes, however, the first step of the evaluation process comes from another family member, or from an observant pediatrician. Sometimes, a child is taken to be evaluated for another disorder, such as Attention Deficit Disorder, and in the process, the accurate diagnosis is arrived at.

Although the pediatrician is an important part of the evaluation team, it's not easy for the child's doctor to pick up signs of Asperger Syndrome in an ordinary well-child visit. However, when parents raise their concerns, pediatricians can guide them toward specialists who can conduct a thorough evaluation.

During the evaluation process, which may take time, you can make an effort to teach social skills more directly, rather than wait for your child to absorb them intuitively. For example, you might look for additional opportunities for your child to play with peers. You might work with your child on ways to approach other children, and practice the phrases that go with this skill ("What are you doing? Can I play?"). This approach would help develop social skills in any child, and would do no harm if your child's diagnosis was fine-tuned later.

Arriving at a Diagnosis

So your pediatrician or someone who works with your child in school has recommended an evaluation for Asperger Syndrome. What can you expect? How can you tell if you're receiving a careful diagnostic evaluation and accurate diagnosis?

Any evaluation, of course, should indicate the extent to which your child's behaviors meet the criteria of the DSM-IV, demonstrating impaired social interaction; impaired communication; and circumscribed, unusual, or repetitive interests and behaviors. Professionals will obtain a thorough developmental history, observe your child in structured and unstructured situations (including during play), review records, and conduct standardized testing for cognitive, social communication, and motor skills.

It is also necessary to rule out other diagnoses that might have been raised as possible explanations for the child's behavior. Does the child show evidence of ADD? Mental retardation? A language disorder? Determining what condition a child does have, and which he does not have, is called differential diagnosis. Some other diagnoses, such as ADD, may coexist with Asperger Syndrome; others, like mental retardation, are far less likely to.

Parents might be asked about the extent of unusual interests or preoccupations, and whether these have changed over time, if they can be interrupted without too much difficulty, or whether the child insists on talking *only* about a particular subject of interest to him.

Like all spectrum disorders, Asperger Syndrome can range from mild to more severe (merging with high-functioning autism). The diagnostic statement should also indicate the severity of each trait. Thus, your child might have great difficulty with nonverbal cues and with social conventions and have an area of intense circumscribed interest, but not show unusual repetitive behaviors. These nuances are an important part of the diagnosis.

All of this should be part of any evaluation for Asperger Syndrome. Beyond that, however, are three elements that are part of a good evaluation.

A good evaluation is holistic. It should be more than a label, or a few test results, or unidimensional measurements. It should be a description of the whole child, including strengths and weaknesses. It should also examine the child's whole environment, looking at how he behaves at home, at school, in the neighborhood, in calm environments, and in stressful settings.

A good evaluation is a team effort. It is not a one-person operation. Although most parents broach their concerns with their child's pediatrician at first, a thorough assessment requires contributions from experts in a variety of fields. It is possible to arrive at a satisfactory diagnosis by consulting one specialist at a time, but that process often means that each specialist evaluates only one aspect of your child, rather than the whole child. Not only can the process be cumbersome and time-consuming, it also runs the risk of less accurately assessing the complex, often subtle manifestations of Asperger Syndrome. For that reason, I believe that it is often advantageous to use an interdisciplinary team approach. Typically, this team is established by professionals who see the child, based upon their initial assessment of areas of need. Over the course of the evaluation, new areas of need might be identified, necessitating the addition of other professionals. By selecting a clinic or program that specializes in the evaluation of children with autism spectrum disorders or Asperger Syndrome, parents can have more confidence that all the professionals needed for their child's team will be included.

The professionals on the evaluation team might include the following:

· *Psychologist.* A psychologist is trained in understanding human behavior and how the mind works. This professional will collect information on your family and your child's experiences within it, including his emotional development, his cognitive abilities, and his social strengths and weaknesses. The psychologist will try to build a complete picture of your child based on observation, interviews, and tests, and will recommend family and educational interventions to help your child. In certain situations, a pediatric neuropsychologist might evaluate your child to gain additional information about specific areas (such as poor memory, poor organizational skills, or evaluation of right hemisphere brain deficits that might indicate a nonverbal learning disability).

· *Physician.* This specialist evaluates your child's general health; assesses his coordination and neurological health, including evidence of seizures; and assesses his motor coordination. Ideally, this doctor should have a special interest in PDDs; a specialty in psychiatry, pediatric neurology, or developmental pediatrics would also be appropriate here.

· *Speech and language pathologists.* This team member will examine your child's facility with language, both in functional terms and in terms of what we call "pragmatics"—the practical and social uses of language. This professional will probably administer several tests of language competence that will determine your child's strengths and weaknesses in understanding and communicating with language.

· *Special education teacher or educational psychologist.* This member conducts achievement tests and determines specific learning disabilities, and also is a key resource in guiding parents toward an educational program for their child.

· *Occupational therapist.* This specialist works with children on assessing and improving the development of fine-motor skills and sensory processing and regulation. This team member also evaluates visual-motor integration, which is important in skills such as handwriting, shoe-tying, and other activities.

While each specialist will examine your child and may write a separate report, the team maintains close contact during the evaluation and contributes to a more unified final report. A case manager serves as your link to the team, so you don't have to approach each specialist separately if you have questions.

Typically, the results of the assessment are presented to you at a meeting called a "parent interpretive." This meeting not only provides and explains your child's diagnosis, but also offers recommendations for treatment, family interventions and approaches, and educational placement for your child.

A good evaluation is prescriptive. It should do more than simply identify and describe your child's deficits. It should tell you what to do about them, and offer specific guidance to others who will work with your child.

In my own practice, I don't let anyone leave my office without a clear explanation of what I recommend be done about each issue raised. I try to give families a template that they can use in a range of

circumstances—if they change schools, for example, the same information would apply in any school setting.

These recommendations should address each area in which the
child is having problems. If the child can't make friends, or has trouble
reading, or other difficulty, we address each area. It's important to
include a description of the child's strengths, as well as weaknesses,
because we can use those strengths to build up the weak areas. If your
child has no friends, but is great at shooting baskets, or memorization,
maybe one can explore athletics or theater as a way to get him involved
in activities with other kids where he'll have a chance to shine.

What Kind of Therapy Is Best for Children with Asperger Syndrome?

Your child's evaluation may include a recommendation for therapy.
Counseling or therapy can be an important part of your child's treatment plan, particularly if he struggles with issues of self-esteem,
depression, or anxiety. However, it's important that any therapeutic
approach take into account the unique aspects of Asperger
Syndrome.

Psychoanalytic therapy—indeed, any approach that calls for
introspection and probing into the subtle or symbolic meaning of
past experience—is likely to be ineffective. As we've seen, people with
Asperger Syndrome have great difficulty understanding and interpreting human emotions and motivations. They are unlikely to recognize or benefit from symbolic or metaphoric interpretations of
behavior.

Therefore, the preferred method is cognitive behavior therapy,
which is more concrete, oriented to the here-and-now, and focuses on
defining problems and deciding how to address them. Children with
Asperger Syndrome tend to be literal-minded, and benefit from a
straightforward, problem-solving approach. Sessions can focus on
trouble spots the child experiences at school, for example, and develop

strategies for coping with them. For children who suffer from depression, anxiety, or panic attacks, drug therapy in combination with cognitive behavioral therapy may be beneficial.

In recent decades great progress has been made in treating, or alleviating, mental and behavioral disorders that had been considered beyond the reach of pharmacology. Conditions such as schizophrenia, bipolar disease, and depression, along with lesser kinds of anxiety and obsessive-compulsive disorders, have been greatly eased by the use of medications that alter and normalize brain chemistry, particularly when combined with effective strategies for teaching the child or adult how to better cope.

Thus, no one can say for sure that drug therapy for PDDs won't become possible. But Asperger Syndrome is related to the fundamental structure and connections within the brain, rather than solely to an imbalance in brain chemistry. At present, there are no studies of psychotropic medications specifically designed for those with Asperger Syndrome. Rather, persons with high-functioning autism, and other PDDs, including Asperger Syndrome, have been lumped together in research protocols. That makes speculation very tentative.

However, certain medications that target difficult symptoms and behaviors associated with Asperger Syndrome have indeed shown promise. For the most part, the symptoms are outgrowths of the fundamental condition: anxiety and depression, for example, that may result from the confusion and frustration that are common in Asperger Syndrome. Some medications that may be prescribed by your child's physician include:

- SSRIs (selective serotonin reuptake inhibitors) such as clomipramine (Luvox), used for depression, obsessive-compulsive symptoms, and anxiety
- stimulants, such as Ritalin, prescribed for inattentiveness
- atypical neuroleptics, such as risperidone (Risperdal), is used for self-injury and aggression, and sometimes for obsessive-compulsive symptoms

- antihypertensives, such as clonidine, and tricyclic antidepressants, such as imipramine, used to alleviate anxiety

Children with Asperger Syndrome have a somewhat higher instance of seizure disorder than do typical children. In these cases, anticonvulsant medications may be advised.

Although these medications can help, many have significant side effects. Both the positive effects and any negative effects of these medications are highly individual; they vary from child to child. That's yet another reason why families of children with Asperger Syndrome must work very closely with the child's psychiatrist or neurologist to monitor the effects of all medications. An in-depth discussion of this complex subject is beyond the scope of this book, but it is important to educate yourself about the medications as you work with your child's medical team. *Straight Talk About Psychiatric Medications for Kids*, by Timothy Wilens (New York: Guilford Press, 1999), is an excellent guide for parents. Ultimately, this decision requires careful assessment by a physician who specializes in treating such problems in people with Asperger Syndrome.

Reacting to the Diagnosis

As we've seen, parents can be devastated by their child's diagnosis. That was certainly true for Ethan's parents, whose story opened this chapter. Yet many parents, particularly those who have had a long, frustrating search for answers, report feeling a profound sense of relief, a sense of finally arriving at a destination.

However, the diagnosis of Asperger Syndrome has implications that go beyond the point of learning the diagnosis. Parents and the children themselves must process a whole range of emotions that come about as a result of this knowledge.

The important thing to remember while you process this new information is to accept your feelings, to face them, and to honor them. Here are some of the familiar reactions that parents report.

Shock and denial. It's quite natural that a parent's initial reaction might be to disbelieve, to reach out for another explanation. To face the reality that one's child has a chronic disability is devastating.

One parent recalls, "When your child is first showing troubling symptoms, you jump to believe what other parents tell you to make you feel better. 'My Johnny never says hello, either.' Or, 'My Janie is shy, too.' You have to resist that."

It's also difficult for parents to face the relationship between Asperger Syndrome and autism, even though the prognosis for Asperger Syndrome is much brighter. "When you learn it's on the autism spectrum, it's overwhelming," one parent recalls. "I wouldn't buy any books on autism. I would only buy books on Asperger Syndrome."

Guilt. It's common for parents to believe that their child's difficulties are their fault. Mothers, in particular, are likely to worry that they ought to have done something differently during their pregnancy, or during their child's early years. "Was it something I ate when I was pregnant? Was it that sip of champagne?" It's also common for parents to look for someone else to blame ("You start scrutinizing your in-laws," said one). Blaming, in itself, is not a constructive emotion. But taking a closer look at the family tree to see if other family members—or the parents themselves—had any traits of Asperger Syndrome or other social/communication problems can be an important part of educating yourself about your child.

Anger. When you learn that your beloved child has a developmental disorder, it is natural to feel anger and resentment. Yet it's difficult to know exactly where to direct that anger—after all, it's nobody's fault. And so parents often go through waves of anger directed at themselves, at the medical and psychological experts who can't "cure" their child, at God, at others who offer words of comfort that don't comfort.

It's not unusual, either, to feel surges of anger and resentment toward children who do not have Asperger Syndrome and their families, for whom everything appears so easy. Even when those children have problems, our reactions can be complex. As one mother recalls, "I get an evil satisfaction out of observing 'typical' children who misbe-have. I know many who tantrum, who can't sit still, and who have poor social skills. My son—now—has better social skills than most kids his age. It was not always this way."

Anger and resentment are not productive emotions, and lead often to shame. (What kind of person am I, you may think, to resent another family for their good fortune? The answer, of course, is that you are a perfectly normal human being who is suffering.) Ultimately, anger is productive if it can be channeled into the energy you'll need as you work for your child's best interest.

Relief. Many parents feel shock and grief at the realization that their child has a disability, yet at the same time feel a great burden lifted from their shoulders because their worries now have a name, a name that suggests a course of action. They have known something wasn't quite as it should be, so the diagnosis offers them a sense of relief and resolution as well as concern.

Renewed focus and determination. If you accept your painful feelings, and give yourself time, you should arrive at a point where you are ready to face your situation head-on. Many parents find that those seemingly negative feelings, such as anger and resentment, can become ingredients of a new kind of energy. Instead of feeling defeated and hopeless, they find within themselves a fierce determination to take on their child's challenges.

"We went from thinking we had a brilliant little boy who could memorize books and videos by heart, to thinking we were in for a life-time of special services for a handicapped child. That's the effect of hearing words like 'Asperger' and 'autism' in association with your child. What we've ended up with is a beautiful, affectionate, intelligent little boy who is now virtually indistinguishable from his peers. Emotionally, however, it's been like bungee jumping."

The important thing to remember while you process this new informa-tion, and work your way through these emotions, is to accept your feelings, even the ones you find uncomfortable. By so doing, you will more easily arrive at the acceptance and resolution that you'll need to move ahead.

It's important to stay close and supportive at this time, and a good way to do that is to be respectful of one another's individual way of processing difficult feelings. Another is to try to meet your spouse halfway on issues where you disagree.

Here are some suggestions that parents have told me are helpful at this stage:

Take time. You and your child will be living with this diagnosis for a lifetime. You don't need to process every piece of information right now, to read every book, to seek every treatment, to take your child to be tested, all this week. Step back, gather your strength, and proceed one day at a time.

Get the facts, but carefully. By reading this book, you are taking the kind of action that will help you and your child. Knowledge is power, and the more you know, the more you can help your child and interpret his needs to others.

However, some of the published literature about these developmental disorders, and autism in particular, are out-of-date, both in terms of treatment recommendations and in terms of the seriousness of the prognosis.

"There's something to be said for not always reading all the literature if it starts making you upset," recalls one mother. "You may start seeing stuff that isn't really there. Your child is the one you have to listen to, first and foremost, and focus on the steps you need to take."

Although Asperger Syndrome is part of the autism spectrum, and some of the same interventions are helpful in both categories, it is essential to focus on the fact that Asperger Syndrome can be much less disabling. A more helpful approach is to read current material on Asperger Syndrome, and to contact the many support sources available on the Internet (see the Resources section and Reading List at the back of this book).

Reach out for support. You have a big job ahead of you, and you'll need help. Help and support come in many forms. Your husband or wife may be your rock, your biggest source of strength. It may be that a sister or old friend who knows how to listen, who makes you feel stronger, is your favored support. There are also many fine organizations (listed in the back of this book) that provide support and information. Most parents report that there is nothing quite as comforting as sharing experiences and concerns with other families who have faced the same challenges—and overcome them.

Take care of yourself. Living with, raising, advocating for a child with a disability is hard work. You need to preserve your health, both physical and emotional. It's not easy to add another "must" to your list, but at least give yourself permission to budget time for yourself, for your relationship, for your exercise and medical checkups. If you are able to schedule it, an occasional dinner out or weekend getaway is not an abandonment of your child, but a good way to build your family's strength for the long haul.

Take care of your relationship. Finally, give attention to your own bond with your spouse or partner. If you are happily married, your spouse most likely will be your strongest supporter, and likewise you will be your partner's best ally. You will need one another now, and all along the journey you and your child take together.

However, raising a child with special needs puts an extra strain on any partnership. Not all relationships are able to withstand the stress. But there are ways to keep your relationship strong during this time. Some couples even report that their child's difficulties bring them closer together and strengthen their bond.

First, recognize that your spouse's adjustment style and timetable may be different from your own. Because you and your spouse are different people, you will have different ways of processing these feelings, and different timetables. You may wear your heart on your sleeve and be outgoing in your sorrow and anxiety, while your partner may be

more introverted and prefer to keep these thoughts and feelings contained. You may read avidly about Asperger Syndrome and join support groups, while your spouse may need to decompress by doing other
things and taking an occasional break from the situation. One of you
may feel the need to consider your child's diagnosis and difficulties a
private matter, while the other may be more open.

Communicate. Although it may be difficult to voice feelings of anger,
despair, or frustration, your relationship will be stronger if you are able to
express your feelings, and accept your partner's. It's normal to feel some
anger and resentment at your spouse. Sometimes that anger originates in
feelings of resentment toward your disabled child—and the thought of
being angry at an innocent child is difficult to acknowledge. Keeping
your emotions bottled up not only adds to your own stress, but keeps you
isolated from the person you need most for support.

Make time together a priority. This means time for just the two of
you, spent doing something enjoyable like having an elegant meal out,
or going to a movie or concert. And don't include your evenings
attending lectures or support groups for Asperger Syndrome in this
category. Those activities are important, but they serve an entirely different purpose. To be strong, your relationship needs and deserves
attention on its own terms.

If you feel your relationship is at risk, seek outside help. Together
or on your own, initiate contact with a couples therapist, preferably
one who has worked with parents of children with disabilities or
chronic illness.

Disclosure: Sharing Your Knowledge with Others

Once you have received your child's diagnosis, the question arises:
What do I do with this information? How do I explain Asperger
Syndrome to my child, my family, my friends?

This process of disclosure about a subject that makes some people uncomfortable is not something you do once and then it's over. You will be explaining and interpreting this condition to others for the rest of your life, and your child will also learn ways of explaining himself to others that suit both the situation and his own needs.

How you explain your child's condition to others, and when (and if), depends a great deal on who those others are and how they respond. You probably are able to assess how your own parents and in-laws will handle the information. Neighbors and friends and casual acquaintances, however, are a different story.

Your child. For many families, disclosure to the child is simple. They simply tell the child the name of the diagnosis, and explain it in age-appropriate terms. Others, however, feel there is no particular need to use the term Asperger Syndrome with a very young child who in all likelihood will derive little meaning from the label itself. Either approach can be fine, as long as the family is comfortable with it. What's important is to concentrate on the areas where he struggles, and point out that there are things that you and he can do about them.

As children grow older, or ask for explanations of their own behavior and the treatments and interventions being used, they should receive more information. Often, Asperger Syndrome can be described as a condition in which children need help and support in social situations because that's the way their brains work. In one family, the parents likened their son's condition, and the special help he received at school, to other children wearing glasses because their eyes needed help to work well.

This functional approach toward explaining Asperger Syndrome to a child tends to minimize his anxiety or worry over the diagnosis. The way you discuss your child's condition with him will evolve as he grows; by the time he reaches adolescence, your discussions with him may address his own feelings and concerns about having Asperger Syndrome.

Your other children. How you explain Asperger Syndrome to your other children depends, of course, on their age. Unless your child's behavior is very disruptive, his younger siblings are likely to adjust reasonably well to his disability. They may, however, notice that their brother or sister "doesn't play fair," or insists on playing "his way" all the time. They can be reassured that the family will work out rules and compromises that protect everyone's rights.

Young children may pick up your own anxiety and concern, and go through many of the same emotional responses you have felt. They may wonder if the condition is contagious. It's important to encourage open discussion of their feelings, to put their worries to rest, and help them realize that even negative emotions are normal and acceptable.

Older children have the advantage of being able to understand what Asperger Syndrome is, and to be supportive in mature ways. A disadvantage is that they are often at a peak of vulnerability about their own shortcomings. They may wonder if they, too, have Asperger Syndrome. They may be concerned about the genetic link, and wonder if their own children might be affected. They may worry about their own negative and resentful feelings toward their sibling. Or they may worry that their peers will mock the oddities of the sibling's behavior.

Other family members. How you explain your child's disability to his grandparents and other relatives depends, of course, on their own personalities and attitudes. It's also important to consider your goals in disclosing the diagnosis. Do you want your relatives to be actively involved in your family and its challenges? Would you prefer that they give you more space? Do you want to help them be close to their grandchild? It may not be possible to reach these goals, but you should consider your own needs, and those of your child, as you discuss this issue with them.

If your family is generally supportive and has been at your side as you have struggled to identify your child's problems, you probably will feel able to explain your child's condition to them openly, and they most likely will continue to be supportive.

Not all families are so fortunate, of course. Even well-meaning family members may deny, or blame, or worry so excessively that they add stress to your lives, rather than give you strength. Others are uncomfortable with disability of any kind. Tensions and hostility within the family make some parents feel the need to maintain distance. In circumstances such as these, parents may opt not to share the diagnosis with family.

You may find a way to garner support if you explain your child's condition in a certain way. One parent who knew her parents would deny Asperger Syndrome, because they weren't familiar with it, told them their grandchild had autism. She felt that was the only way to get through to them and get them to face the gravity of the situation.

Another parent said, "My mother is in complete denial. Even today, when my son does or says something that is completely appropriate, she will glance at me in an accusing way, as if I am making all this up."

It's also possible to disclose the symptoms in general terms, without the label, if you think that's better. Just as you might do with your child's siblings, you are explaining the condition in functional terms—in terms of things he is able to do well and things he has trouble with, rather than in terms of labels.

Friends and neighbors. As with grandparents and family members, denial is a common reaction among adults. Family may deny because they find it difficult to face the implications of a disability. Others tend to deny because they haven't heard of Asperger Syndrome; therefore, they conclude it doesn't exist.

For many families, the most comfortable approach is to tell others that their child has a learning disability that affects his ability to know how to behave socially. For others, and for those in a supportive setting, full disclosure is the best route. We'll discuss strategies for explaining your child's behavior and needs to others in your neighborhood and community in chapter 6.

Sharing the diagnosis with your child's peers is a sensitive issue, because so much depends on how those children and classmates have been taught to respond to people with differences and disabilities. In some settings, teasing is almost the norm. Other children may make fun not only of your child's behavior, but of the name of the condition ("Asparagus," "Ass Burger," "Hamburger," and the like). If you sense that sharing the diagnosis will make things harder, rather than better, for your child, it may be best to avoid using the label, and describe your child's condition as a learning disability. "It's hard for John to understand what people mean unless they say it clearly," you can say. "That's the way his brain works."

In other settings, children do well at understanding and supporting a child with a different way of perceiving and learning. We'll discuss more on how to help other kids understand and support your child later on.

Becoming Your Child's Advocate

As you educate yourself and others about your child's disability, you are beginning the first steps toward becoming your child's advocate—a role that will evolve as your child grows. From your first stunned responses at your parent interpretive meeting, to your child's conferences at school, to your efforts to put appropriate adult and community services in place, advocacy is a lifelong process. You will represent your child's interests in many settings. You will be your child's ally and champion, and you will become the model for your child advocating on his own behalf as an adult. We'll come back to your role as advocate in later chapters.

4

The Thunderstorm Prison

How It Feels to Have Asperger Syndrome

Even when he was a very small child, sudden noises terrified Eddie, causing an inescapable terror despite the most soothing intentions of his attentive but confused parents. Rain hurt his ears. Thunder, in particular, caused his heart to race. Other noises, especially unexpected ones, upset him: the whirring of the electric can opener, the hum and whoosh of the vacuum cleaner and his mother's hair dryer, the sudden start-up of his father's lawn mower. These were Eddie's private enemies, at once devastating and understood by few. It was several years before he learned that he could control some of these sounds, and the terror they imposed, by his own means.

The little boy who learned to cry with fright when the sky darkened during daytime also taught himself to read weather maps by the age of four. With their predictable black patterns against white, isobars became his source of comfort as well as a window to information.

By the age of ten Eddie had decided to become a meteorologist. He had amassed a wealth of information about weather patterns and phenomena, sharing it with anyone who showed even the slightest interest or inclination. After writing a letter to the local television meteorologist, he became the weather spotter for his community, reporting on temperature, wind velocity, and other weather conditions whenever called upon.

While the Weather Channel became his lifeline to facts and phenomena around the globe, it also became a harbinger of those things that terrified him the most. Like the barometer he so assiduously watched, his emotions rose and fell with his ability to predict thunderstorms. He knew that thunderstorms followed a somewhat predictable pattern of occurrence and severity throughout the year, and tracking them became an obsession.

Somehow, the predictability of knowing that a thunderstorm was approaching, or even likely, allowed him sufficient time to collect himself and prepare emotionally for the noise. At most, Eddie would broach the subject frequently with his parents, pester them with questions about whether they thought a storm was probable or only possible, and then retreat to his silent preparations. After the storm had passed, Eddie would record its occurrence in his log book, checking it against the expected average for that time of the year. Most times, this strategy worked.

But sometimes it did not work. It seems that August is peak thunderstorm season where Eddie lives, with, on average, four days with thunderstorms. By August 15 one year there had been none, and when the mild weather continued into the third and fourth weeks of August, his sense of foreboding grew. By August 26, alarm was turning to panic at the probable violation of an otherwise predictable—and safe—rule. His fear that there would be fewer than expected thunderstorms in August was compounded by his belief that any one of them could be more sudden and violent as a result. His parents' efforts to explain the fallacy of his thinking did little to assuage those fears. On August 28 his panic reached its peak as he realized that there could not be four days with thunderstorms by month's end. The pacing and repetitive question-asking about the storms that started slowly at mid-month reached a fever pitch.

Then came September, and with it, relief. School was starting, and Eddie's worries about August's averages were eleven months away.

To the outside observer, Eddie's interest in meteorology and thunderstorms might appear to be an obsession, pure and simple. But it is much more: in addition to being a genuine fascination, it is a lifeline. Like many people with Asperger Syndrome, Eddie's area of interest provides him with a whole array of rituals that help him control his anxieties.

The need for predictability is a hallmark of Asperger Syndrome, and immersing oneself in a narrow subject is immensely soothing—until the unpredictable happens. When August goes by without thunderstorms, the familiar reliability of weather projections loses its ability to calm Eddie's fears.

To the unenlightened observer, a child like Eddie has a hobby, and simply needs to branch out into other areas of interest. His parents might decide to enroll Eddie in summer camp, or pressure him to take up golf during the summer to help him loosen his grip on his obsession with weather. But such a course of action could be just the wrong approach. While there is wisdom in helping Eddie broaden his interests, it's essential that those who wish to help him understand his behavior from his perspective—from the inside out.

The mechanism of Eddie's behavior begins with his sensitive hearing, which is not unusual for people with Asperger Syndrome. Loud noises hurt, and sudden loud noises both hurt and startle. It's stressful to know that you're going to be startled, and not know when. Thus, learning to predict the kind of thing that upsets you is immensely calming.

In this chapter, we'll examine the behavior of children with

Asperger Syndrome from their perspective. Then we'll pinpoint how to apply that knowledge to your dealings with your child. We'll try to help you feel what your child is feeling, and what lies behind the behavior that sets your child apart from typical children. Once you have that insight, you will feel less confused and baffled by her behavior, and you'll be able to guide and help her.

If you've put yourself in her skin, you can feel how itchy that particular blouse feels. If you walk in her shoes, you can feel where they pinch. If you understand how she sees and hears and processes sensory input, you can anticipate the buildup of tension she feels at the mall, the airport, the neighborhood street fair. If you understand that she processes language in a very literal way, you can adjust the way you speak to her.

In short, knowledge and insight will help you be more supportive, and enable you to offer appropriate guidance. Without it, you run the risk of being less empathic, and are more likely to apply interventions that will only confuse her more.

One wonderful resource for insights into the mind of people with autism spectrum disorders is Temple Grandin, a writer and professor who is a world authority in livestock management. Over the years I have been privileged to spend time with her presenting at conferences, and discussing her experiences in academia and as an individual with an autism spectrum disorder.

As a young child, she was diagnosed as having high-functioning autism, and she often describes herself that way. Certainly in early childhood she was much more severely impaired than most children with Asperger Syndrome. Recently, however, she has wondered whether, as an adult, her symptoms overlap with Asperger Syndrome. She clearly falls within that area of diagnostic overlap we discussed earlier, but whatever the label, her insights provide a window into the world of many people with Asperger Syndrome.

Grandin's books and lectures provide useful insights into how she felt growing up, and how she responded to sensory events (scratchy clothes, physical closeness) that she found frightening, painful, and confusing. Her memories and insights are similar to those that my patients have discussed with me, both as children and as adults looking back on their lives.

Grandin's earliest memories are of fear, confusion, and frustration at her inability to make sense of her world. As a small child, she reacted to this confusion by exploding into violent tantrums, or alternatively, withdrawing into soothing rituals.

"I could sit on the beach for hours dribbling sand through my fingers and fashioning miniature mountains," she writes in her autobiography, *Emergence: Labeled Autistic*. "Each particle of sand intrigued me as though I were a scientist looking through a microscope. Other times I scrutinized each line in my finger, following one as if it were a road on a map."

She also took refuge in spinning, either spinning herself or spinning other objects. Watching the world spin around her as she twirled, she felt a sense of power and control. Watching other objects spin gave her a sense of tranquillity and serenity, and helped to block out sounds that caused her distress. "Intensely preoccupied with the movement of the spinning coin or lid, I saw or heard nothing. People around me were transparent. And no sound intruded on my fixation. It was as if I were deaf."

Of course, many children twirl themselves around and fiddle with simple objects. But for children with autistic spectrum disorders, this kind of ritualistic behavior provides more than amusement.

Let's look at the ways people with Asperger Syndrome perceive the world. Not every child has all these perceptions, but you are likely to find your child somewhere in the following descriptions. Then, we'll discuss what you can do with that information to help your child.

Sensory Overload and Integration of Sensory Information

Most of us pay little attention to our own senses. Our eyes and ears and skin bring us information; our bodies perceive temperature and pressure in ways we can easily process. If we're cold, we put on a sweater, and that's that. But for children with Asperger Syndrome, senses provide unreliable information at best, and discomfort and anxiety at worst.

We all vary widely in the sensitivity of our senses—the sharpness of our hearing, our visual acuity and sensitivity to light, the intensity of our sense of smell and taste, and the degree to which we can detect changes in temperature, pressure, and the other information that comes through our sense of touch. These normal variations contribute to our many talents. A chef with a fine sense of flavor, or a musician with perfect pitch, is admired.

But sometimes heightened senses, or hypersensitivity, can be an inconvenience, and more. If you are a princess in a fairy tale, it may be difficult to find a comfortable mattress. If you are a child with Asperger Syndrome, you may have difficulty shutting out annoying sounds and aromas. Although not all children have this trait (it is not required for a diagnosis of Asperger Syndrome under DSM-IV), it is common.

In addition, children with Asperger Syndrome may experience hyposensitivity, or reduced or lessened sensitivity, in some situations, and seek unusual amounts of stimulation. It may be that some of the self-stimulation characteristic of children with autistic spectrum disorders—fidgeting, rocking, or spinning of oneself or objects—is related to a need for more sensory input.

The term "sensory integration dysfunction" has been used to describe difficulty that many people (not all with Asperger Syndrome) have with modulating and regulating sensory input. Although the scientific evidence supporting sensory integration issues as a disorder is inconclusive, it's helpful to look at this approach as we try to understand and help children with Asperger Syndrome cope adaptively.

Sensory integration refers to the process that typical people manage to do quite effortlessly: take in messages from the senses, integrate them into meaningful information, and use them to formulate appropriate responses. When this process is not working well, difficulties arise in concentration, physical movement, and the ability to formulate appropriate responses to the environment.

In addition to the basic senses of hearing, vision, smell, and touch, the brain also must process information that comes from within the body: the vestibular sense, which provides information about movement, gravity, and balance; and the proprioceptive sense, which communicates messages about body position and body parts. Both these senses are important in physical coordination. When they are well developed and functioning as they should, they convey a sense of ease and confidence in movement that help the child play and explore with grace and freedom. When these senses are poorly integrated, a child may move awkwardly, or may be fearful of participating in activities in which she feels off-balance.

The integration of sensory information is also important in the brain's efforts to attune to the important messages, and tune out the unimportant ones, or those to which we've become habituated. Thus, most children are able to pay attention to a puppet show and ignore their body's signal that the chair is hard and uncomfortable. Or the child may become accustomed to the distracting sound of an air conditioner, and "learn" to ignore it. When sensory integration is not working well, incoming sensations jostle for attention, and the child has great difficulty selecting the important messages, attending to them, and paying less attention to the unimportant ones.

For example, a child who approaches a group of girls jumping rope on a hot summer day might have difficulty in many areas: she might be so distracted by the uncomfortable sensations of heat and humidity that she has difficulty concentrating on social skills such as approaching the girls and asking to join in. Or if she does participate, her sensory difficulties might make the coordination in jumping rope nearly impossible.

Let's look at the basic senses and examine how sensory difficulties can make life difficult for people with Asperger Syndrome.

Hearing. As we've described, Eddie had particular difficulty with hypersensitive hearing. When he was a child, the noise of thunderstorms overwhelmed him. Many noises that typical people simply tune out are highly distressing to people with Asperger Syndrome. Often, they are shrill or high-pitched sounds, like those made by hair dryers, blenders, and vacuum cleaners. When those noises are sudden or unpredictable (as thunderstorms were for Eddie at the beginning), the discomfort is augmented by fear and panic.

Auditory sensitivity may mean the ability to hear sounds that others can't, from a conversation in the hall outside the classroom to the sound of one's own heartbeat. It also can mean feeling distress at noises that others hear but don't find distressing—the whooshing sound of the wind in an open car window, for example.

One mother I know is organizing a social group of middle-school boys with Asperger Syndrome. As the five boys gathered in the den in her home, they had a hard time settling down; they wanted to find out what was making "that noise" they all heard. "That noise" turned out to be the faint hum of a water cooler that nobody else could hear.

This sensitivity can also result in difficulty processing sounds, especially in conversation. People with Asperger Syndrome may have difficulty following conversations, sorting out one voice from another—and even more trouble figuring out the emotional meaning of people's tone of voice.

Sudden sounds, and sounds that convey a sense of danger or uncertainty, can be particularly distressing. The ringing of a telephone startles many people with Asperger Syndrome, partly because it happens without warning, but also because it signals the beginning of a social interaction that may be challenging.

School fire drills can be both painful and frightening for children with Asperger Syndrome; there's the sudden loud ringing, followed by the tension of everyone scrambling out of the classroom, and the unexpected change in the day's routine. And then there's the emotional aspect of the situation (is it a real fire this time?). Children who cry, or cover their ears, during fire drills may be chastised by teachers and teased by classmates, all of which increases their dread of future fire drills.

Vision. Children with Asperger Syndrome may have normal vision, but find it difficult to process certain stimuli, such as bright lights. The beach can be a source of stress on many levels—along with scratchy sand and stinging salt water, there's the harsh glare of the sun. High contrast between light and dark may be uncomfortable or distracting.

Fluorescent lights are a particular problem because they flicker on and off at a rate most people are unable to detect. Some people with Asperger Syndrome may perceive them as brightly flashing lights, a considerable distraction. If your child is bothered by these lights, it will be difficult for her to concentrate in a classroom where they are used.

This sensitivity can go two ways: certain stimuli may be distressing, while others may having a calming effect. Children may become entranced by moving lights or objects that others wouldn't notice—the sparkling reflections from an icicle, or the swirling colors on the surface of a puddle in the street may hold their attention for long periods of time.

Smell and taste. One of my patients can smell nail polish on his mother's fingers for days after she has a manicure; another can walk into an office or store and tell that it has been repainted, even when the redecoration occurred weeks ago. This same child became ill on his kindergarten class trip to an apple orchard; the smell of the old cider press that everyone else found pleasant and atmospheric was too much for him.

Your own child may also be able to detect faint odors that others can't, or may be overwhelmed by stronger odors. She may have finicky eating habits, because some foods upset her—slimy foods, hard foods, "noisy" food that crunches. The color of certain foods may be upsetting, or she may take comfort in eating only foods of a particular color.

Touch. For many children, an acute sense of touch translates into difficulties with clothing. Scratchy labels, tight shoes or neckties, prickly wool socks—all may generate feelings of discomfort that lead to difficulties with dressing and clothing selection. Socks with seams are a source of discomfort for many kids. Many typical children exhibit these sensitivities as well, but children with Asperger Syndrome perceive these discomforts as pain, or as sources of panic.

Temple Grandin describes how much she hated having to get washed and dressed; having her hair shampooed was painful, as if the person rubbing her head had thimbles on her fingers. Dress-up clothes, especially petticoats, felt like sandpaper against her legs. She also recalls how much she dreaded being hugged, even by people she was fond of. She particularly disliked it when affectionate relatives would come visiting, and swoop down on her with their engulfing embraces.

Temperature can be a source of discomfort and often leads to conflict. A child who suffers when overdressed in the winter may be reprimanded for refusing to wear a jacket. Or bath water that parents think is pleasantly warm may be perceived as scalding to a child. Some children with Asperger Syndrome experience pain from ordinary bumps and pokes that seem insignificant to others, but other children seem to experience no pain when they are hurt quite badly.

Because children with Asperger Syndrome may experience individual senses with more intensity, they may have more trouble than most people taking in all this input and making a coherent whole of it. In the typical brain, sound and sight and smell are processed smoothly; a conversation with another person involves integrating the other person's words, spoken volume and intonation, perfume, and the meaning of their words. To the child with Asperger Syndrome, it may be difficult to concentrate on all these issues at once. As we'll see, when sensory overstimulation builds to a crisis point, the result runs the gamut of troublesome behaviors: withdrawal, anxiety, ritualized behavior, or outright tantrums.

How This Information Helps You

We'll offer specific suggestions in later chapters, but the key point, as it relates to understanding your child's feelings, is this: Sensory overload is real, and it's important to acknowledge your child's feelings.

However, as with all the aspects of Asperger Syndrome that contribute to unusual behavior, your child will have to learn to modify some of her reactions. Even a child with intensely felt senses cannot stay wrapped in a blanket or under water for her whole life, nor can she expect the rest of the world to come to a halt as it accommodates her sensitivities. Thus, compromise is called for.

As we'll illustrate in later chapters, there are ways that your child can learn to buffer herself where possible (comfortable clothing, for example) on one hand, and extend her comfort zone on the other. The feelings may be real, but what a child does about them can be managed in creative ways. For example, you can allow her to wear comfortable clothing, within reason. But you can also encourage her to stretch herself in some settings. For example, she might come with the family to the fireworks display, but be permitted to wear ear plugs or wait some distance away where the noise isn't so loud.

Your willingness to help, to offer acceptable compromises, does several things: it decreases her discomfort, it helps her expand her range, and it demonstrates to her that you understand and are on her side.

Impaired Communication

Remember Ethan, the boy with a rigid fixation on train schedules? When his mother talked about the importance of being flexible, he retorted that pipe cleaners were flexible; how could people be? Or David, whose teacher thought he was being sassy when he responded to her requests with a studied literalism?

Such responses are typical of the way a child with Asperger Syndrome uses and hears language. Language is literal to such a child. It serves to organize facts, and to convey information. The use of idiom and metaphor are difficult concepts, and while they can be learned to some extent, it is like learning a foreign language. "Why can't people say what they mean?" my patients ask me.

The child with Asperger Syndrome may feel left out of conversations because of this, and may further withdraw from confusing social situations. Later, older children and adolescents get quite fed up. "Why can't people be logical?" they grumble. During the teen years, slang phrases and vocabulary become an important part of social conversation. Imagine the effect on a literal-minded child with Asperger Syndrome when a classmate expresses delight and disbelief with the phrase, "Get OUTTA here!" She may take the words literally, reacting with hurt, anger, or both.

Another area of difficulty is what we call paraverbals. These are nonspoken cues, like body language, that are enormously important in conveying meaning in face-to-face conversations. They vary from culture to culture, but most people learn them without effort. For example, we all follow unwritten rules about how close we stand next to a conversational partner. While speaking with an employer or someone we don't know well, we all naturally tend to stand about an arm's length from that person. With a spouse, however, we stand much closer. It's easy for someone who hasn't learned these rules to make social errors, and to offend others without realizing it.

These unspoken rules include the rhythm of language. A group of people conversing has a musical quality that most of us learn "by ear." We join seamlessly into a conversation. We generally have a feeling for when to laugh out loud, when to smile, when to nod, when it's our turn to speak, when it's appropriate to interrupt.

Interrupting, by the way, is a highly refined skill that most people learn quite effectively. If you listen to a conversation among a group of friends or acquaintances, you'll observe that people often don't finish a sentence or thought completely; others jump in with their own comments quite frequently. Technically, they are interrupting the speaker, and yet they aren't being rude. These interruptions keep a lively conversation moving forward, and actually add to what the speaker was saying by providing quick examples or details that show interest. Interrupting is offensive when it is poorly timed or changes the subject entirely, a conversational faux pas made frequently by people with Asperger Syndrome.

And then there are what we call metamessages—for example, expressions of polite disinterest versus active disinterest. People with Asperger Syndrome have trouble with the emotional content of language; they may not recognize a tone of voice that signals sarcasm, or the sighs and fidgets that tell the speaker his story has gone on too long. By the same token, they may not pick up on signals that convey someone's interest: the eager, interested facial expression, or the frequent nods of agreement.

Sometimes the other aspects of Asperger Syndrome, such as ritualized behavior or unusual interests, are used inappropriately in conversation as inappropriate bids for social interaction. If you're not a particularly good conversationalist, it can be tempting to stick to an area where you feel competent. One patient of mine used to ask me, and everyone else he came in contact with, for their license plate number (of course, he knew mine by heart, from repeated queries). He did this because it constituted a "conversation starter" for him; whenever he used it, people would usually pay attention, at least for a moment.

All these aspects of communication—the spoken language and the nonverbal body language, not to mention appropriate topic selection—constitute the pragmatics of language. The pragmatic rules guide us as we try to communicate our intended message to another, and as we try to determine what another person's message is. We have to understand and follow these rules in order to tell when someone is teasing, being polite, or being sarcastic.

When you think about what goes into language and communication, it's quite amazing that most of us handle this complex system as well as we do. It helps to have some sympathy for people who aren't at ease with this complexity.

We all have to learn these rules, of course, but most of us learn them quite early. By the age of four, most children can take into account the setting or context of their conversation, and adjust their speech accordingly. They speak differently to adults and teachers than they do to a younger child. They clarify their messages, ask others for clarification, and show the beginnings of self-censorship in certain situations. For example, at three, a typical child riding the bus might ask loudly, "Why that lady so fat?" At four, she may ask the same question, but in a whisper.

How This Information Helps You

The child with Asperger Syndrome does not learn these rules through osmosis; you will have to teach your child the rules of communication in a much more overt manner than you would your other children. One of the most effective ways of doing this is through rehearsing and scripting. Before a bus ride, for example, you can state some rules ("We sit down in an empty seat, but we don't sit right next to someone if there are lots of empty seats. We talk quietly . . .").

As you become more aware of how your child processes language, you will see how difficult it is for her to keep up with ordinary conversations, and you'll be reminded why it's important to keep your explanations and verbal instructions straightforward and to the point. You will make an effort to speak clearly and plainly, to avoid metaphor and idiom, or at least to explain it when you use it.

Impaired Social Interaction

Asperger Syndrome is characterized by a lack of awareness of many aspects of social behavior. And yet most people with Asperger Syndrome are aware of their lack of awareness. They may realize that other people seem to understand the nuances of life, but they don't understand how those others do it.

A typical problem of social interaction is not knowing how much importance to put on a particular aspect of someone else's behavior. Overinterpretation of social behavior is a problem. A teenager is accidentally jostled at a crowded mall, and interprets the jostle as an act of aggression. She may respond aggressively, with dire consequences.

Overinterpretation is particularly troublesome when ambiguous nonverbal behavior—a hearty slap on the back, for example—is combined with ambiguous language ("What's the matter? Cat got your tongue?").

Underinterpretation is the flip side of the same issue. When your listener starts looking at her watch, it means you have gone on too long in your one-sided conversation and ought to wind it up. But that cue is frequently missed. Or a teenage girl riding the subway may not realize that the man who is sitting too close isn't being truly friendly.

Adolescents, in particular, suffer from this sense of not understanding what's going on. So much of "normal adolescence" (if there is such a thing!) involves paying close attention to peer norms and subtle distinctions between groups and individuals as one tries to find one's place. The teenager with Asperger Syndrome may be preoccupied with how to fit in, and think that if she just tries harder, approaches the problem more logically, she might succeed. Some, who are justly proud of their intellectual abilities, declare that they don't have friends because "Everyone else is stupid." It's an attitude that doesn't help their cause. (We'll discuss the experiences of adolescents with Asperger Syndrome in chapter 9.)

A mother who hosts a group of middle-school kids with Asperger Syndrome says, "Most children are not reflective enough until they reach adulthood to really understand the lifelong implications of their Asperger Syndrome. They seem to understand bits and pieces—kids don't like them, they have trouble with anxiety, they have good memories—but I don't think they understand the total impact that this will have on their lives."

As we mentioned in the context of sensory overload, the difficulties that kids with Asperger Syndrome have in social interactions can cause great stress, especially as they grow older. Tension, nervousness, and "fight-or-flight" responses are common. Children may withdraw, take refuge in ritualized behavior like fidgeting or flapping, experience panic attacks, or lash out in anger.

How This Information Helps You

As we discussed above, your child needs to learn the rules that govern spoken and unspoken language. In the same way, you'll need to help your child learn the specific social skills that will serve her well. You will have to teach her the rules: when it's OK to pick your nose, and when it's not. You'll instruct her in such matters as how to approach an acquaintance, wait her turn, or line up at the water fountain.

Brenda Smith Myles refers to this as the "hidden social curriculum." As you help explain this curriculum to your child, you should also convey your sympathy for how difficult it is for her and your recognition of how hard she is trying. Eventually, your child probably will be able to develop considerable insight into her own behavior, and identify how it is different from typical behavior. She'll be able to sense that she's made an error, and begin to work on ways to avoid repeating it. It's a useful skill to develop, and one that you can help your child learn. As we'll discuss in later chapters, there are techniques you and your children can work on together that continue this process of examining her difficulties and learning new strategies from them.

Repetitive or Unusual Interests and Behavior

As we observed with Eddie, an intense interest in weather and thunderstorms has a meaning much deeper than meteorology. Eddie uses the intricate details of his chosen field as a source of comfort and calm.

Many children with Asperger Syndrome exhibit similar retreats and rituals. Whether it's weather or train schedules, their focus on the area of interest increases when they feel greater stress.

One mother reports that she worried when her son told her that he reads voraciously "to escape reality." She worried that he was expressing a profound sadness, or dissatisfaction with his life. Later, the family was at a noisy restaurant, and he clearly became upset at the noise. He began to shake his head sideways, as if to get water out of his ears. His mother told him to stop, but he said, "Mom, the noise is really hurting me, and I'm trying to clear my head—to shake it out. This is why I need a book, to escape reality."

At that point, his mother realized that his "escape" reading wasn't so much a psychological need, but a physical, sensory one. He was able to tune out stressful sounds and reduce his anxiety when immersed in a book.

How This Information Helps You

Often, the odd behaviors you observe are your child's attempts to cope with her unusual senses, reactions, and perceptions. She is struggling to ease discomfort, and is being resourceful, on one level. What looks odd on the outside is doing its job; she is easing her stress in ways she has discovered are effective.

When those methods bring her negative responses, you and she will want to work on ways to change them into more acceptable techniques. But the starting point for this is to honor what she has accomplished.

If you understand what's behind your child's fidgets, routines, and immersive interests, you are empowered in two ways: First, an increase in such behavior signals that your child is feeling confused or anxious. Second, you can work with her on coming to some sensible compromise about how much of her time is devoted to a particular interest. Ethan's parents, you'll recall, issued "train schedule tickets" that permitted, but limited, his obsessive checking of train schedules. You'll come up with similar strategies that allow your child the comfort and security of ritual and routine, but that begin to set some parameters on it. Again, we'll discuss this more in later chapters.

A Self-Assessment

"I don't like being labeled with Asperger Syndrome, because it makes me sound like I'm retarded. Even though I know I'm smart, and even though my classmates and teachers know I'm smart, people who only know about the Asperger Syndrome before meeting me don't know that. They treat me like I'm stupid and dependent. It can be very frustrating. I don't like to think of myself as having Asperger Syndrome. I think that basically I'm a normal kid, except I think about things more. I ponder life and the world. This gives me a different view than most people, and makes me smarter."

This young man, a former patient of mine who is entering an honors undergraduate program at a major university this fall, is able to appreciate his own strengths. He knows how, and in what areas, he is smart. He has learned, as have many people with Asperger Syndrome, how to assess others' opinions of him. He bristles at unjust assumptions that others may make about him. Although this process of figuring out other people and their state of mind is more laborious for him than for typical people, he is able to do it.

He has correctly assessed his own strengths: He is a focused, logical thinker in a world where such thinking isn't exactly the norm. His condition requires him to be more thoughtful about everything, since he can't rely on intuition. He "ponders life and the world."

Your child, too, is working to figure out the world, its wonders and complexities, and to establish her place in it. She is doing this from her own quite remarkable perspective, and it's different from the way the rest of us perceive our world.

Your child's senses—sight, hearing, and touch—may be different, or interpreted differently. Her understanding of spoken language and body language is different. Her choices of activities and interests are made differently. The more you are able to understand your child's perspective, the more you will be able to offer her guidance, interpret confusing situations, and help her build her skills. And all the while, you'll stand side by side, enjoying her company and cheering on her successes.

Part Two

Asperger Syndrome
and Your Child

5

The Wordless Lullaby
of Airplanes

Your Child Within the Family

The sound of an approaching airplane always pleased him. Even before he could speak, the distant drone of propellers and the soft roar of a jet caused him to look upward, pointing excitedly. No one in the family was surprised when he said his first word, "airplane," before he reached one year.

As John grew, his vocabulary skills and reading ability expanded quickly. Words soon became sentences, and sentences long soliloquies about many things of interest to him, but mostly airplanes. He didn't notice that his interest confused his classmates, or caused them to go home from play dates prematurely. His parents, both puzzled and proud of their son's knowledge, wondered whether this interest would lead to a future in aviation or engineering. No one doubted the child's intelligence; he had always been clever, and then some. But that single-mindedness! John would either grow up to be a very determined young man, or a genius appreciated by only a few. Those possibilities worried his parents.

Living on the flight path of a major metropolitan airport

gave John many opportunities to expand his knowledge of airplanes. In addition to learning about maps and geography, he
mastered the silhouettes of airplanes in flight. Much as his classmates would learn to identify dinosaurs and animals, he would
commit to memory the profiles of 727s, DC-9s, and the various
fighter planes hangered at the adjacent Air Force Reserve airfield.
Adults were often amazed at his impressive fund of knowledge.
His classmates, however, often were less amused.

John's ability to discern sounds was as sharp and focused as
his visual perception of dark shapes against a sky. Soon the differences between engines made by Pratt and Whitney and those made
by Rolls-Royce were as obvious to him as the different cries of a
baby are to a mother. He could now be soothed in the darkness of
his room at night by the approaching planes.

As he progressed up through the elementary grades, John's
social awkwardness only became more evident. Not that he didn't
have friends; several other children along the way shared some of
his interests. But these liaisons lasted only as long as the interests
coincided. Once gone, the friendships drifted.

He became upset sometimes at things considered trivial to
others. The bell at a fire drill, the whine of the kitchen blender, or
the change in his daily schedule at school could send him into a
panic. He felt trapped and powerless, without plan or recourse.
And then John discovered that he could soothe himself by creating
the sounds of airplane engines. Like a wordless lullaby, he could
drone those sounds, and reduce his fear in minutes. The strategy
was effective, but not always appreciated. His teachers discouraged
it while his classmates and neighbors looked askance at him. His
mother never condoned it, but she understood.

Returning home from high school quite agitated one afternoon, he soon began to hum the sounds. The din and pitch escalated,
as did his pacing throughout the halls of the house. John's resourceful mother gave him a tape recorder and sent him to the basement to
record his own airplane noises. He returned thirty minutes later,

calmed. The tape recorder gave John a ready-made audience and an alternative source of engine sounds all in one neat, portable package. It gave his mother a needed respite from his mantra.

Headphones made the ritual more private, and also more acceptable. Well-made tapes he saved for future use. He learned to structure his use of the noises to calm himself around those times when he had his tape player and headphones in hand, and his panic became more a matter of self-control. Maintaining a tape player with his daily effects was an easy, efficient strategy. As he entered adulthood, and got a job, the tapes went along. Almost no one who worked with him knew why the tape recorder was present, but everyone knew that he liked it.

And yes, John still can spot a P-38 in flight as it overflies the crowd during the September air show.

As John's story suggests, Asperger Syndrome has effects that go beyond the child himself. Parents, siblings, and other relatives become aware of a child's differences, put up with annoying behavior, appreciate unusual talents, and ultimately—if they are wise—pull together to find ways to help the child grow and develop.

And that, of course, is what families everywhere do. As you observe the behaviors that set your child apart from typical children, and as you work through your reaction to your child's diagnosis, it will be tempting to focus so much on the differences between your family and other families that you forget the ways in which you are similar. It's easy to become so attuned to the challenges you and your child face that you forget that you'd still have difficulties if your child did not have Asperger Syndrome.

In this chapter, we'll look at how your child with Asperger Syndrome fits into your family, how you can support and encourage him, and how you can structure family life so all its members are nurtured and feel a sense of belonging. Because later chapters deal with the developmental issues affecting older children, this chapter will focus primarily, but not exclusively, on young children.

Let's begin with a "mission statement" about all families, with and without a disability.

You Are a Family First

It's true that you have a child with a disability, and this will effect everyone in your family in numerous ways. But you're still a family, the same people you were before you learned of your child's condition. That doesn't change. The strengths and attachments that bonded you before are still present.

Families are about belonging. Ideally, they provide a place where every member is accepted and respected, where every member's needs are met, and every member's contributions are expected and honored.

Families are made up of individuals who vary greatly in their needs and ability to contribute. When children are young, they need immense amounts of nurturing and effort and patience, and it's usually the adults who make the greatest contributions. Over time, as children become stronger and more independent, this balance shifts somewhat. Eventually, the oldest family members may count on assistance from younger members.

This variation isn't limited to age, of course. If a family member has special needs, those needs must be met as well.

But it's important to remember that everyone in your family has important needs, not just the child with Asperger Syndrome. So as you organize your family life to best help your child, you'll need to keep sight of the fact that your other children, your spouse, and you yourself need the support that family brings.

The Asperger Syndrome Family Dynamic

Every family operates under a system of "rules" that, though often unspoken, are understood and usually (but not always) obeyed.

Although some families have better sets of rules than others, the rules usually bring a certain order, predictability, and security to everyone's life.

They can be minor, like who sits where at the dinner table. You don't have to use place cards; all the family members know where they belong. They can be major, like who handles most of the child care and who earns income outside the home.

As time passes and circumstances change, the rules need to be revised. A new baby unsettles the routine. The family moves to a new house. There may be divorce or death. A child leaves the nest and goes off to college.

In families with a child with Asperger Syndrome, the dynamic takes a particular form:

Diagnosis. In one sense, you became a family with Asperger Syndrome at the moment you learned of your child's condition. But in another sense, you began to make subtle adjustments long before this, as soon as you detected areas in which your child was "different." If your child has been extremely sensitive to particular noises, you have probably been adjusting to that for some time. Perhaps you can only use the hair dryer when your child is out of the house, or use the power mower when he's at school.

Your child's diagnosis further disrupted your family dynamic and made it necessary for you to revise some of the rules in order to cope with new demands. You also have been coping with your emotional responses to the diagnosis. You have no doubt been learning what you can about Asperger Syndrome and working to ensure that your child gets the appropriate services and interventions.

Accommodation. Once your child is diagnosed, the accommodations you may have made all along become clearer. You may have had to adjust your work schedule, or your social obligations, to accommodate these responsibilities. New "rules" come into play. You carefully maintain routines so as not to upset your child. You learn what kind of clothing is most comfortable. If your child is often out of control behaviorally, you may stop having friends over for dinner. Family decisions about holidays and vacations may be made around the child's needs.

Definition of roles. As the family accommodates to the child, members take on defined roles. Mom may be the school advocate and Asperger Syndrome expert; Dad may supervise homework. One parent may consistently be the one who attends to the child's outbursts, always leaving the movie theater or the restaurant when there's a scene. One older sibling may provide babysitting, while another has the role of playing and socializing with the child with Asperger Syndrome.

Crisis and redefining of rules and roles. Every family evolves, and children grow, become teenagers, and leave home. These are natural "crisis points" that are followed by an unsettled period. Other crises are less predictable. The family moves. A parent or grandparent dies. Parents divorce or remarry. In all these situations, the crisis is followed by a disruption in routine until family members establish new rules and define their new roles.

Other crisis points occur when the child with Asperger Syndrome makes a developmental leap, such as beginning school or moving from elementary school into the adolescent stresses of middle school. But there can be subtle crisis points when other family members achieve developmental milestones—confirmation or bar mitzvah, going to the prom, getting accepted at college. These moments in family life can draw attention to the fact that the child with Asperger Syndrome isn't keeping pace.

The cycle continues throughout life. It's normal for the rules to adjust at each point. But sometimes families don't adjust smoothly, or fail to adjust at all, when circumstances call for change. Although rules and routines help stabilize and bring security to family life, there is a danger in sticking to rules that have become outmoded. If no crisis stirs up change, we have a tendency to stick with what works.

Sometimes we fail to pay attention to the growth and development that makes change necessary. As your young child learns to dress himself, for example, you'll change your routine to recognize his progress. As your child learns social skills, you'll be able to adjust your own schedule and social life accordingly.

Indeed, when your child makes progress, that calls for more than just a change in routine or a sigh of relief. It calls for praise and celebration. Take advantage of every forward step that your child takes as a teaching opportunity. Whether you give a specific word of praise, a gold star on a chart, a high-five, or a special outing or celebration, make it clear that you are proud of your child, that he has made great progress, and that he can look forward to more such milestones.

Your Other Children

If you have more than one child, you will no doubt worry about how your child with Asperger Syndrome will influence the family, and specifically how your other children will be affected. And you are right to think that they *will* be affected.

Any disability brings with it challenges for family members. A child with Asperger Syndrome may behave in ways that are inappropriate or intrusive, and provoke more disputes and fighting than in typical families. All this can put a strain on the entire family, and calls for greater levels of supervision.

However, this does not mean that the effects on your children will all be negative. Yes, the whole family will have to adjust, but many siblings of children with disabilities rise to the occasion. They may squabble and complain about their sibling, but they may also play joyously, provide useful insights, and become fierce advocates for their brother or sister.

That does not mean that they must be selfless saints. You would worry if they were. What they will be are brothers and sisters. They will be themselves.

And your child with Asperger Syndrome is a brother or sister *first*. As such, he will do things to annoy his siblings. He will drive them crazy. He will be perceived as getting unfair advantages. That should hardly be surprising. *All* children complain about their siblings in these ways, whether that sibling has a disability or not.

Your task, as parents, is to meet the needs of all your children, which is no small order. But this means not only allowing your other children to have their own lives, apart from Asperger Syndrome, but helping them feel comfortable and at home with their feelings—both positive and negative—about their sibling.

For example, if your nine-year-old complains that her seven-year-old brother is refusing to cooperate when they try to play together, you can say, "James has trouble playing school with you because you are creative and like to make funny and interesting things happen in the class. Just now, you made him be the teacher and you were the student. When you make up surprises, he's so set on following the rules that he can't figure out what to do. He's fine when you are the teacher, and you keep things the same, or else explain it to him when you do something new."

This perspective allows his brothers and sisters to take an educative approach—to teach him how to behave. Enlist your other children as members of the team that's going to help James figure out how to behave.

Remind your other children that they're going to feel annoyed at times, and fed up, and that not only is this normal, it's universal among all families, whether there's a disability or not. Their feelings need validation, just as yours do (as we discussed in chapter 3).

For the most part, older siblings of children with Asperger Syndrome can be quite cooperative and protective, especially when they have a good understanding of the disorder. I've seen brothers and sisters intervene in social settings and either divert teasing before it starts or protect their sibling if things get out of hand.

Protectiveness sometimes declines when the sibling becomes a teenager and becomes intensely sensitive about "fitting in." Having a sibling with this disability can be an embarrassment at times. Often when this happens, it's a signal that older siblings need more space, time away from the child with Asperger Syndrome, to develop their own lives as adolescents. They are likely to become more supportive over time, as they become more mature and confident.

A caution: As helpful as your other children might be, be careful to avoid becoming overly dependent on them for support. If your older child is missing out on his teenage social life because you expect him to babysit during your evening shift at work, you will want to rethink your arrangements. Your other children can be enormously supportive of their sibling with Asperger Syndrome, but they are entitled to their own lives as well.

Structuring Family Life

The family is the ideal training ground for children to learn the skills they'll take with them into the community, the school, and beyond. Let's look at some ways to make your family life workable, and to use these early years to your child's advantage.

There may be times when you despair of having a calm, "normal" family life. Perhaps your child has frequent tantrums, or you struggle to schedule your grocery shopping because he can behave only for short periods of time. At such times, it may be helpful to remember that most families' lives are not particularly calm. You may not achieve the ideal you have in your mind's eye, but you can ensure that your family performs its function: providing nurturing and support for all its members and guiding them toward independence. You have more control over how things are handled in your own family than you do in other spheres, and this control is an advantage as you structure your home for the benefit of all its members.

Below are what I call the Golden Rules for survival in families with a child who has Asperger Syndrome.

Predictability. All children do best when they know what to expect. But for your child with Asperger Syndrome, predictability is a lifeline.

You have probably observed this trait in your child, such as when you learn that, year after year, your child memorizes the names of classmates and their assigned seats within the first week of school. You've probably also witnessed its excess, when your child is totally upset by any unexpected event.

An organized family life is not easy to achieve, but you can strive for it. Prepare your child for changes in routine, and use calendars, clocks, and timers to help illustrate to your child when some event will occur. Some small children may be reassured by simple explanations of what the day has in store ("First we'll go to grandma's, then we'll stop at the library. Then we'll come home and have grilled cheese sandwiches for lunch."). Others might need this sequence written down or described with a picture schedule.

One family uses a calendar with extra-large blocks to map out the family's week. Each member's appointments and activities are written in a different color ink. For eight-year-old Carlos, red ink signifies his activities. His school day is marked as a block. Appointments are indicated in the appropriate day. Carlos can see not only his own schedule, but those of other family members as well.

Before the calendar system, Carlos used to become upset when his father traveled on business. But now, he can see the dates clearly on the calendar, predict his father's departure, and anticipate his return.

If the family is planning a vacation trip, you and your child might cut out pictures from magazines or travel brochures to illustrate the places the family will visit. An older child may take an interest in charting the itinerary on a map. Share the planning and preparation for the trip with your child, including lists of what to pack.

Of course, the best-laid plans often have to change. Whether it's a flat tire, a delayed flight, a sudden snowstorm, or a case of the flu, unforeseen events force schedules to change. This is an area of great difficulty for children with Asperger Syndrome, but they can adjust. Carlos becomes upset when events don't match the calendar perfectly, but he's learning to cope if he's given ample warning. If you know ahead of time that something has been rescheduled, inform your child ahead of the change.

Last-minute changes in schedule are the most difficult. Your child may get upset when plans change at the last minute. Later in this chapter, we'll discuss ways to help your child become more flexible.

Structure. Unstructured time can be Dante's tenth circle of Hell. Your child with Asperger Syndrome has great difficulty structuring his own time and behavior, so when structure is not imposed upon him, all sorts of breakdowns occur. The capacity to self-structure is related to executive function, as we discussed in chapter 2. It requires the ability to plan, and to impose order on a random environment. Recess at school is often a difficult time, because there's no clear script for behavior. Sensory overload, growing anxiety, and tantrums and out-bursts may occur as a result. Your task at home is to ensure that your child has a clear understanding of what to do during the day, including playtime, chores, homework, and other activities.

Lists and schedules and, again, calendars, can be used to help your child know what to do when. A clock or kitchen timer can alert him to transitions from one activity to another. You and your child can construct a schedule for school mornings that takes him through every step, from waking up to heading out the door with his backpack.

Your child can have a weekend schedule that outlines his free-time activities in detail: television time, breakfast, chores, lessons, quiet time for reading or computer, games or outdoor play with brothers and sisters, and so on. It's wise to review the schedules with your child, include his input if he desires, and have him practice following the schedule and making the transitions from one activity to another.

Routine. A clear understanding of what the family does when, and a consistency in that schedule, will be your most useful tool in organiz-ing your child with Asperger Syndrome within the family. A routine provides both predictability and structure, and your child will usually be eager to comply.

Now here are two more rules, which we'll call the Silver Rules for survival.

Responsibility. Remember that all family members should pull their weight—according to their ability. Contributing to the well-being of the family is important on two levels: it lays the groundwork for skills that lead to independence, and it provides a sense of pride and accomplishment. Don't allow protectiveness to deprive your child of these benefits. Do remember, however, that chores should be assigned according to ability, rather than to the inherent usefulness of the task. When a small child helps get dinner ready, that assistance may actually delay the process, but it's still an important lesson. Gradually, the child's help becomes more effective, and important lessons in responsibility are learned.

However, the issue of chores has to be worked out according to your child's unique circumstances. The stress and anxiety of getting through the school day can leave some children with Asperger Syndrome with little energy left for chores—or for dealing with additional demands from parents. Be sure to select a responsibility that is within your child's power to accomplish, and do what you can to avoid making it an additional level of stress in your family.

Children with Asperger Syndrome often enjoy taking on responsibilities for tasks that are done the same way: setting the table, feeding the dog morning and night, or putting their dirty clothes in the hamper.

Keeping one's room clean is a responsibility that may or may not be easy for a child with Asperger Syndrome. For every child who is orderly and meticulous, with everything in its place, there's another who is so disorganized that room-cleaning seems an overwhelming project.

With fairly complex tasks, such as room cleaning, it's a good idea to break the job down into parts and assign one part at a time. Or you can set priorities. Perhaps your child can manage part of the room responsibility—like making the bed, or keeping laundry off the floor—

but not the entire project. For the big picture, it's helpful to take a Polaroid picture of the room when it's clean, and post it so that your child can see what a good job should look like.

Here are some other tasks that your child might perform that build a sense of responsibility without being overwhelming:

· watering plants
· bringing in the newspapers
· putting groceries away in the pantry
· emptying the dishwasher and putting things away
· feeding pets
· folding laundry
· doing "research" for the family (looking up words in the diction-ary, places in the atlas, weather information on the Internet, and so on)
· calculating gas mileage on a trip

Tasks that promote ultimate independence are best. When you are at the grocery store, your child might be able to get items from the gro-cery list. He might have difficulty selecting the best produce, but he might be a whiz at collecting the canned soup and boxed cereal on the list. Chores like this serve several purposes: the child performs helpful work, develops his own abilities and confidence, and learns important skills that he'll need later in life.

Flexibility. Almost any task that your child performs—whether in the category of household chores, schoolwork, or other activities—offers him the opportunity to develop flexibility.

The ability to roll with the punches and readjust when circum-stances change is an important ability, but one that's usually lacking in children with Asperger Syndrome. It can be taught, however. You can teach your child specific rules for what to do when something happens that wasn't on the agenda. I call these "What-if?" exercises. You can ask, "What should you do if you come home and there's nobody here?" or "What should you do if the door's locked and nobody's home?"

You and your child can brainstorm answers together, tossing out ideas and then selecting the best response. Some answers might be: Watch TV and wait for Mommy or Daddy. Find all the cookies and eat them. Go next door and tell Mrs. Baxter. And so forth.

After you've collected several responses, you can evaluate them. Eating all the cookies may not be the best approach, but the other two options have merit. Help your child select the best choice.

Of course, the nature of the unpredictable is that it's unpredictable. You may have taught your child what to do if nobody's home, but what if there's been a thunderstorm and a big tree is blocking the street? Who can plan for every eventuality?

The answer is that you can't, but you can branch out from your flexibility rules toward more global critical thinking. Ask your child "what if" from time to time. Mix in some familiar scenarios to which he knows the answer, along with some new ones.

For example, you might say, "What if we go to the deli to buy the kind of potato salad you like, but they've run out?" You and your child can discuss various options: pick some other flavor, go to another store, give up, and so on. Model how to select options from a menu of choices.

Always praise your child when he remembers an established "what-if" rule, or when he comes up with good options in new situations. Praise, also, when he demonstrates willingness to be flexible or to vary from a rigid routine.

One reason it's a good idea to involve your child in these "What-if?" activities is that he will need, eventually, to make decisions in a whole realm of situations. No matter how specific your instruction is, you will not want your child to be overly compliant in life. It's important for him to have some experience making choices, being in control, and saying "no." The ability to speak up, state one's wishes, and refuse requests some of the time is essential to your child's well-being.

It will be an important element in his personal safety later in his life, as well.

Coping with Specific Asperger Syndrome Issues

Let's examine some ways to approach your child's behavior that relates specifically to Asperger Syndrome.

Sensory issues. We've described the sensory discomforts that children with Asperger Syndrome frequently exhibit. Family life can certainly be disrupted when other members are constantly accommodating themselves to the sensory issues of the child. But there are ways to ease these disruptions, and help your child be comfortable as well. The key is to accommodate the sensitivity, where reasonable, and try to expand your child's tolerance, when necessary.

Thus, once you understand the source of your child's need for soft, nonbinding clothing, you will all get along better if you accommodate that need. Once you find out what your child is comfortable wearing, it may be wise to purchase several sizes to accommodate growth.

There may be times when it is reasonable to seek compromise, however, or to try to expand your child's tolerance. On special occasions where everyone will be dressed up, your daughter's choices aren't limited to a crinkly party dress that would make her miserable, or her usual faded sweat suit, which wouldn't be appropriate. She might wear "dress-up" comfortable clothes, such as a colorful jumper and cotton leggings. Your son might wear a soft cotton sweater over his usual T-shirt. Or, for a really formal occasion, your child might have to wear the uncomfortable clothing for a while, but you might take along a change of clothing for him to slip into once the main event is over.

Many children with Asperger Syndrome have difficulty with clothing fasteners, in part due to their motor difficulties, and also possibly because of sensory sensitivity. Buttons, for example, can feel lumpy against the skin, and also can be difficult to fasten and unfasten. Clothing without buttons and zippers may be preferable, although your child should be encouraged to learn practical dressing skills.

Sometimes occasions that make children uncomfortable have inherent rewards that can be used to lure them into tolerating more experiences. Your child may enjoy collecting shells at the beach, but dislike scratchy sand and stinging saltwater. He may love the appearance of the fireworks, for example, but be terrified of the sound.

Andrew, for example, responded with pain and terror to the Fourth of July celebration as an infant. The family's outings to the park would end in misery when the fireworks began and Andrew had to be taken home, much to the displeasure of his sister. But Andrew did like the idea of watching the fireworks, so in later years he was provided with earplugs, and he and his father watched the display from the distant parking lot. Each year, they moved closer, and now that Andrew is eleven, he enjoys the holiday festivities fully.

The lesson here is not that all children with Asperger Syndrome will enjoy fireworks, nor that enjoying them is an essential life skill. But it demonstrates how the technique of accommodating the discomfort, and expanding the level of tolerance, can make it possible for kids with Asperger Syndrome to tolerate many more activities.

You can apply this approach to other realms. Your child can wear sunglasses or visors if glare is a problem at the beach, and over time work his way out from under the umbrella and toward the waves.

When food is an issue because of flavor, aroma, or texture, it may be wise to accommodate up to a point, but to introduce new foods gradually. Even when your child retains his strong dislikes, he can learn to express them politely and refuse food graciously. A fussy eater who can say, "No, thank you," is more pleasant to be around than a fussy eater who announces, "Eeeww! This stinks!"

It's also important to reward progress. Thus, if your child is able to stay in the same room with you while you vacuum the rugs, when last year he covered his ears and cried, he has made progress that should be acknowledged. Similarly, if he comes up with a solution to help him cope with a sensory issue better (as John did, with his airplane noises), you should praise him for his creative and sensible approach toward coping with discomforts.

Interestingly, although your child's hypersensitivity is likely to continue, it may moderate in time. Some experts say that people with Asperger Syndrome either experience less sensitivity as they grow older, or they learn ways to cope with it.

Intense interests. Coping with the intense interests and questioning of a child with Asperger Syndrome can be wearing in itself. It is also worrying, since we sense that the child would benefit from a bit more flexibility.

But as we've seen, children with Asperger Syndrome are often enormously persistent in their devotion to their favorite subjects. John's parents had little hope of diverting his interest away from airplanes, and most parents likewise find that their child's focus is more than an interest or hobby; it's a lifeline. They look for ways to allow their child the comfort of the special interest in a way that allows some growth and flexibility.

Tony Attwood, an Australian psychologist who specializes in Asperger Syndrome, has developed these suggestions, based on two techniques: controlling access to the interest, and finding ways to apply the interest constructively.

If your child is devoted to butterflies, you can develop a system under which he can pursue the interest—with certain limits. For example, you and he can establish a certain amount of time during which he is permitted to work on his butterfly collection, and set a timer for the end of that period. When the timer rings, he must switch to another activity, perhaps a favorite computer game. At that point, he must either move to another room, or the equipment for the hobby must be removed, to help reduce temptation. The activity he switches to should be another pleasurable one and not be perceived as a punishment.

Controlled access can also set up a positive system of rewards. For example, compliance with household rules and expectations for a certain amount of time can earn him another book on butterflies or a collecting expedition.

It's never too early to look for ways to help your child use his interest constructively. Constructive application means, first of all, that you look for ways that your child's intense interest can be a strength. As he grows older, the opportunities increase—in school, he may gain recognition for his excellent science project on butterflies. Or, with other interests, he may become the school computer or chess wizard, and make friends that way. In later life, his area of focus may open up career opportunities.

Constructive application of the interest might include using an interest in maps and national flags to learn about current events, or baseball teams to learn U.S. geography. A child who is a whiz at computers can be genuinely helpful as the family's "technical support" person. Your young meteorologist can keep track of when frost is forecast, and take responsibility for bringing the hanging plants inside on cold nights. By being creative, you can help relate your child's interest to other subjects or tasks.

Later, you'll learn ways to help your child use his special interest to attract and maintain social interactions. We'll discuss this potential further in the next chapter.

Building basic social skills. As we've said, the family is the ideal place to nurture beginning social skills. All children need to be taught how to behave appropriately in social situations, and the family is the first teacher.

A typical child will absorb social learning almost effortlessly, by imitation and positive reinforcement. At age two, he'll offer a guest refreshment by extending a crumbled cookie in his hand. His parents praise his hospitable impulse, even as they sweep up the crumbs. Later, he offers juice to a friend who's come over for a play date.

Other skills are taught more explicitly, such as when to say "please" and "thank you," and what conversational topics are acceptable in various social settings.

But children with Asperger Syndrome need much more direct instruction in social rules and expectations. Here are some essential skills that children with Asperger Syndrome should be developing in the family setting:

· Making polite greetings and responses.
· Refraining from hitting or poking.
· Making requests and expressing desires in an appropriate way. This might mean asking for something with words, rather than grabbing or screaming.
· Sharing and taking turns. Sharing is not an easy skill for children with Asperger Syndrome to learn (in fact, it's difficult for most children), but it's really the underlying rule for many social activities. When you take turns playing a game or using a toy, that's sharing. And when you engage in social conversation, that's sharing, too.
· Following basic rules of conversation. Young children can practice making eye contact, at least part of the time, listening, pausing for the other person's response, and so on.
· Interpreting. If your child can copy your behavior, or imitate a facial expression, it will help him better interpret the social intentions of others.
· Initiating play (approaching a group of children and asking to join in).
· Understanding degrees of intimacy and the appropriate language for each. Children need to learn that behavior appropriate for the family is different from behavior appropriate for public settings.

Following are some techniques that you can use to help your child acquire these skills in a family setting:

· Be explicit and specific whenever you instruct your child. If your preschool child screams whenever he wants juice, you will have to explain that screaming is not allowed, but give him appropriate language to use instead ("May I have some juice?"). An older child can learn the specifics of introductions and greetings: ("You hold your right hand out, smile, and say, 'Hello, Mr. McCarthy' ").

· Encourage your child to observe other people's social signals. For example, you can say, "Your sister is sad because her friend moved away. See how her mouth isn't smiling?" He may not be able to understand right away, but gradually he will learn to read these.

· Use pictures or drawings to draw your child's attention to facial expressions or body language. You can practice with pictures of faces that are smiling, sad, angry, and so forth.

· Teach your child the appropriate words for emotions, and the behaviors and facial expressions that tell us what emotions others are experiencing. This is the first step in helping your child recognize his own emotions. He may know, for example, that he feels a tightness in his throat when he feels bad about something; it may take him a while to associate that physical feeling with the word "sad."

· Teach the proper ways to behave with different people. What's OK for family isn't necessarily OK for strangers (although little kids get more latitude). Draw a picture of concentric circles: family in the middle, then relatives, friends, acquaintances, and strangers. You can discuss what greetings are appropriate for people in different levels of intimacy, what kinds of behavior are suitable for relaxed at-home time with the family, and what kinds of behavior are necessary when one is out in public.

· Practice skills with your child. If your child tends to avoid another person's gaze, you can ask him to look at you for a moment and say "Hello." You can have your child approach another child (using a sibling, if necessary) and practice phrases like, "May I have a turn?" He can practice knocking on a sibling's door and saying, "May I come in?" rather than barging in uninvited.

· Practice suitable ways to initiate conversation. For very young children, such phrases as "What are you doing?" and "What's your name?" can go a long way.

· Encourage flexibility. Once your child has mastered a rule (for example, if he has learned two or three conversation openers), try expanding his knowledge or varying the situation slightly. To further develop flexibility and generalization, you can apply the "What-if?" techniques we discussed earlier to social skills. For example: "What if you say, 'What are you playing?', and the other children invite you to play, but you don't know how to play that game?"

· Reward and praise your child when he learns a new skill or makes progress. And reward and praise when your child cooperates with your efforts to teach him. Although some children with Asperger Syndrome may resist, most respond to clearly defined rules and can be encouraged to cooperate.

If you have other children, your child has a great opportunity to learn essential skills from them. You'll have to structure the rules of engagement, however, so that your other children understand the ground rules. No teasing or taunting, for example. And older siblings will be much more willing to cooperate if they understand how their sibling with Asperger Syndrome learns and what underlies his behavior.

You can explain to your other children why it's hard for the other child to understand what's expected, or why it's so hard for him to share, or to stop doing an activity that he is enjoying.

Encourage group play at least some of the time, but do honor your other children's needs for respite, for time of their own, and for time and space to play with their own friends unmolested by annoying siblings.

Grooming and hygiene. Along with social skills and basic etiquette, you will also need to teach your child the basic rules about public and private behavior—his own and that of others. Much of this can be done in the context of grooming and hygiene; for example, your child will need to know that going to the toilet and bathing are usually done in private, and that one does not enter bathrooms when someone is using them.

As you teach basic grooming skills, such as bathing and hair combing, keep the tone specific and relaxed. It's an easy way to introduce the essential lessons about sexuality, which will have to be approached in a way that is honest and specific. It's best to teach your child the correct terminology for genitalia and other body parts. Typical children are able to pick up an amazing array of synonyms (including euphemisms and slang) for body parts and functions, and learn which situations to use them in. Children with Asperger Syndrome are less likely to figure all this out, so they're better off knowing the correct, grown-up words from the beginning.

In addition, you'll want to teach your child the specifics of "good touch" and "bad touch"—the rules about where other people may touch a child (on the head, shoulder, etc.) and where they should not (parts covered by a bathing suit, for example). Much of the curriculum that teaches children personal safety relies on interpreting feelings (some touches make you feel uncomfortable; others make you feel happy). Children with Asperger Syndrome may have difficulty with such subtleties, and are better served by specific rules.

As always, tell your child to report any inappropriate or confusing behavior to you or his teacher. He should be able to come to you for interpretation of many kinds of situations, not just in the realm of personal safety.

Discipline

Discipline is not the same as punishment. Good discipline for all children is educative; it tells them how to behave well and be rewarded for good behavior. Establishing appropriate limits and helping children manage their own behavior is essential both for children's development and for keeping a home that's tolerable for everyone in the family to live in.

For the most part, your child's behavior will depend more on his comfort level than on his intrinsic goodness or badness. Most outbursts and inappropriate behavior result from anxiety and confusion. Thus, you can go a long way toward helping your child behave by paying close attention to his setting, his routines, and his anxiety levels.

Conventional wisdom about discipline these days leans away from simply telling children what to do, and toward letting them learn through consequences. Thus, there may be a rule about being home by dinner time; if Alex fails to show up or call to explain his lateness, the consequence is that he can't go out the next afternoon. For most children, this approach is sensible because it permits them to learn by experience. They dislike the negative consequences, and apply that knowledge to their behavior.

When the child has Asperger Syndrome, however, your approach has to be more explicit and overt. Your child likely has difficulty figuring out correct or appropriate behavior from a real situation, and has trouble anticipating likely consequences. You need to tell your child quite plainly what to do, rather than expect him to "catch on" the way typical children might do.

Also, although rules are your friends, don't become enamored of rules for their own sake. Try to limit rules to those that serve a functional purpose—safety, civility, a pleasant home life—rather than focusing on more abstract ideas of obedience and compliance.

Techniques That Help Kids with Asperger Syndrome Manage Their Behavior

The following are what I like to call the Four Cs of discipline techniques that are likely to be helpful with children with Asperger Syndrome.

Be clear. Suppose you are at the mall with your seven-year-old, and you're going to have to walk through the store's china department in order to reach the exit. You worry about your child running off, bumping into tables, touching the china, or other potential disasters. If you say, "Behave yourself in the store," he won't get a clear picture. Instead, you'll need to say, "Hold my hand, and don't touch the things in the store. They break easily."

It's also good to try to phrase rules as Do's, where possible, along with Don'ts. For example, "Don't play in the street" is essential, but you can include the positive side: "Do play in the back yard." And remember to compliment your child when he complies with a rule.

Be concise. In that store full of breakables, you can say, "No running. Stay by my side." Long explanations with strings of cause and effect are difficult for any child to learn from, and especially so for a child with Asperger Syndrome. What you wouldn't say in the store, for example, is, "If you run in the store, you might bump into a table and the expensive china would break and they'd be mad and Mommy would have to pay for it and we wouldn't be able to buy a boat and Daddy would be mad and . . ." Your child would be unlikely to gain useful guidance from such a presentation. It's great to point out causes and effects, but not at the expense of brevity.

Be consistent. It's essential that your expectations remain reliably consistent. If kids are allowed to bring food into the family room, but not the living room, that rule needs to be enforced consistently. That means you'll have to be vigilant, although your child may well take on the role of enforcer—for his siblings.

Use consequences. Misbehavior should carry a predictable consequence. Although children with Asperger Syndrome may have a more difficult time learning from consequences alone, they are often capable of seeing the link between the violation of a rule and the consequence for the violation. If your child knows the rule against eating in the living room, and the consequence (having to vacuum the living room rug), then the consequence should be imposed reliably when the rule is violated.

Consequences for misbehavior should be selected with care. Clearly, they should be reasonable and clear. But they also should be "negative," meaning that they should discourage the inappropriate behavior, not encourage it. Thus, a child who violates rules about poking and hitting may be seeking attention, but using inappropriate means toward that end. If you make a production out of the occasion, you may be rewarding inappropriate attention seeking. Conversely, for a child whose favorite activity is being alone with his computer in his room, a time-out in his room may not be an appropriate consequence.

It's also wise to probe the causes for violations of behavior rules. If you ask vaguely, "Why did you do that?" or even "What's the matter?" your child may not be able to explain his feelings clearly. It may be more useful to talk about what happened that might have upset his routine. Ask specific questions such as "Are you angry because it's time to turn off the television?" Usually, a behavior problem occurs not because your child wants to be bad, but because of a breakdown in predictability, structure, or routine. Fixing that breakdown often will improve behavior.

For example, a change in household routines can cause confusion. If you have a rule against eating in the living room, your child may follow it without difficulty. But if guests come to visit and are allowed to "violate" the rule, he may become upset and have a tantrum.

Techniques to Avoid

·   Physical punishment. Generally, physical punishment is not advisable for any child. For a child with a disability related to understanding the social signals of other people, this is particularly inappropriate.

·   Screaming and yelling. As we've seen, children with Asperger Syndrome are often oversensitive to noise, and are susceptible to anxiety. Although most parents occasionally become upset and raise their voices, it's not an effective way of helping a child make sense of what he is expected to do.

·   Put-downs, insults, or sarcasm.

·   Overuse of time-out as a consequence. Sometimes a "voluntary" or "personal" time-out is useful for a child who is becoming stressed. But as we've said, sending a child who prefers being alone to his room may not be effective.

·   Subtle consequences. Suppose you tell your child that if he leaves his Legos all over the floor, some will get lost and later on he won't be able to find them when he wants to build something. That may be true, but it's unlikely that he will apply that knowledge and pick up his Legos. It's better to tell him clearly that he must put the toys back.

·   Long-winded lectures. Keep your discussion of rules and consequences short and to the point.

·   Sulking or other indirect expressions of displeasure. If your child has displeased you or behaved poorly, you'll need to say so. He will not be able to pick up on subtle expressions of disappointment or hurt feelings on your part.

Your child really is trying to figure out what to do. Build on this by telling him what to do, so he can behave well and earn your praise, rather than be reprimanded for misbehavior. And when he does do well, be sure to acknowledge him promptly and explicitly.

Remember that good discipline educates. It tells the child what to do differently next time, so he can be praised for better behavior instead of reprimanded for inappropriate behavior.

The Thrill of Rules, the Agony of Mistakes

Not only are specific rules and guidelines the only way to teach behavior, they also are welcomed—even revered—by the child with Asperger Syndrome. Rules are generally easy for the child to remember, and they offer much-cherished order to the world. That doesn't mean they'll always be obeyed, however. Thus, there must be a system of consequences for shortfalls, as with any system of discipline.

And finally, remember that errors will always occur, mistakes will be made, and your child will have lapses. As you follow through with consequences, also use these errors as learning opportunities. Use what I call "Oops!" strategies. "Oops!" is what we say when we make a mistake. Everyone does it, and everyone has to say "oops" once in a while. Remind your child that like everyone, there will be times when things don't go well, or when rules get forgotten. The thing to do is learn from the error, discuss it, and figure out a way to avoid it in the future.

Ultimately, that's what families are for. They're a safe place to learn, to try, sometimes to fail, and to learn from our errors. Once your child gets out into the big, cold world, the stakes get higher. But if he's begun the learning process at home, his tasks will be less daunting. In the next chapter, we'll examine what your child needs as he ventures out beyond the nurturing, protected environment of his family.

6

The Wedged and the Winners

Integrating Your Child into the Community

At the Presidio's Letterman Gym, a group of ten- and eleven-year-old boys is engaged in basketball drills. They are members of the basketball team of Claire Lilienthal, a public K–8 school in San Francisco. Off to the side, one of the boys from the team is running in strange patterns, laughing to himself, oblivious to the drills. That boy is our son, William.

William has a form of autism known as Asperger Syndrome. It is characterized by a combination of high intelligence in some areas with strange perseverative behaviors, awkwardness in social interactions and speech, and often a lack of physical coordination.

By no means has William achieved in athletics what I had hoped for him several years ago. But he enjoys being on the team and is slowly showing improvement. His gains are due, in good part, to the enormous change in attitudes on the part of coaches and other children over the past decade . . .

In recent years, William has participated on the various

school teams: soccer in the fall, basketball in the winter, baseball in the spring. Claire Lilienthal has an ethos of inclusiveness, so that all children are encouraged to participate. Coaches rotate players, and all players get significant playing time....

In basketball, we practice regularly before the season, shooting, dribbling and passing... As soon as team practice starts, William's reflexes are far too slow for him to be competitive. In the basketball games, he gets on the court and wanders about, often trailing the action, several steps behind. In the first six games, he touches the ball only one or two times, and only for short passes. Still, he likes being on the team and looks forward to the games.

In the early 1960s, when I was William's age, forms of autism and other neuro-developmental disorders went largely undiagnosed. The kids were considered strange or weird or out of it. They had little interaction with other kids, or were teased or bullied.

Today, I'm amazed at how William's classmates treat him. Some teasing occurs, but more commonly they encourage him, support him, include him. At basketball practice, they make sure he gets at least a few touches and direct him back to the game when he starts to wander around. This spirit of inclusion allows kids like William to achieve far more than they could before...

A few weeks ago, the Lilienthal basketball team had its final league game. The coach sent William in for a second time late in the game. Since Lilienthal led its opponent, Presidio Hill, by 16 points, parents and spectators were only paying half attention, talking among themselves.

As the time clock was running down, though, one of his teammates dribbled the ball over to William near half-court. The other teammates on the court formed a type of wedge toward the basket, as they shouted to William to dribble to the basket. After hesitating, William did so until he got to within a few feet of the basket.

Suddenly, the gym became quieter. As the teammates

shouted, "Shoot, shoot," William sent the ball up in his unortho-
dox underhand style. The ball rattled around and then dropped in,
a moment or so before the horn sounded. Silence, and then parents from both teams and the referee cheered loudly. The other
Lilienthal boys came to give him high-fives, and he ran to me saying, "I made a basket. I finally made a basket."

Always a winner.

Your child is not just a part of your family. Your child with Asperger
Syndrome is also part of a larger community. Whether it's your apartment building or your street or your city's recreation department, the
community can be your child's staunch supporter, as it is for William,
whose father wrote this story for the *San Francisco Chronicle*.

But building that kind of support and encouragement from the
world beyond your own family does not happen automatically. It's a
process, and whether you realize it or not, you have been involved in it
for some time already.

From the first time you explain your child's behavior or diagnosis
to neighbors, or when you teach your child at home to dress herself
and say "please" and "thank you," you are working toward the day
when your child will draw confidence from a greater community than
you, as a family, can provide.

In this chapter, we'll discuss that process of moving out from
beyond the comforting sanctuary of home. And we'll focus on the two
areas where you have a crucial role: First, you will need to help your
child build social skills appropriate to the settings where she'll find
herself. And second, your child will benefit if you can become an advocate for your child in the community—both in finding and supporting
appropriate activities, as William's parents did, and in educating others
about the needs of children with Asperger Syndrome. For William's
family, the avenue into community was athletics. For other families,
that avenue might be music, art, religious organizations, Scouts, vol-
unteerism, or something else.

We'll look at young children who are in the beginning stages of making their way into the community from the sanctuary of family, and are relating to others outside the family on a regular basis—children through the first year or so of elementary school, or to about age seven or eight. These years contain your child's earliest forays out into the world of play dates, walking the dog by herself and greeting neighbors, or standing in line at the ice cream stand. She'll answer the telephone, answer the door, begin music or swimming lessons, and attend religious services—sometime with you, sometimes on her own. Children with Asperger Syndrome often develop later than typical children when it comes to friendship issues and interacting with their peer group. We'll save those issues for chapter 8, which will examine the social and communication challenges experienced by children as they move through elementary school.

These are pivotal years for all children, of course, and much trial and error goes on. If your five-year-old wanders into your neighbor's house uninvited, you may feel embarrassed and apologetic, but you can rest assured that countless five-year-olds throughout history have done the same thing.

Just as home and family provide some protection as children learn the rudiments of social behavior in their earliest years, your young child with Asperger Syndrome still has time to learn; you and your child have a kind of safety net during these years. That's because nobody really expects perfect behavior or flawless social skills in a very young child.

These years are, thus, the ideal time to help children build specific skills, their understanding, and their comfort levels. The standards will get higher as the years go by.

So Many Skills, So Little Time

If you set about to teach your child everything she'll need to know in life, the task is daunting indeed. Where does one begin? How can one anticipate every possible skill, and have the time to teach it? There are no easy answers, but there are some ways of approaching the problem that help. I should mention that there are curricula available that do a fine job of providing a core of social skills for children, and which you might wish to (see Skillstreaming curricula by Research Press, in the Bibliography for chapter 6).

What works best with children with Asperger Syndrome is to look at everyday situations and determine what's needed in each of these. Rather than just teach an assortment of skills, and hope that your child will apply them appropriately in the real setting, it's important to see what skills are necessary in individual settings.

Of course it's obvious that particular settings call for particular skills. Buying something at a convenience store may mean only that you behave in the store and be able to place your purchase and your money on the counter. But if you buy your treat at a traditional candy counter, you have to tell the clerk what you want and how much.

We'll discuss these issues in terms of what's called ecological inventory a careful determination of what the particular environment requires. Setting is crucial in influencing the kinds of skills your child will need, and the kinds of flexibility that she'll have to work on.

An ecological inventory simply asks what is needed in a particular setting or activity for the child to do well. It amounts to a list of skills and behaviors that can be clearly defined and explicitly taught.

But because children with Asperger Syndrome have difficulty generalizing—that is, applying one set of skills to a new setting—you may have to teach a set of skills for each new setting that your child is likely to be in. You could teach your child the importance of sitting politely, and waiting to be offered food when she's visiting Great-Aunt Eleanor, but she might be completely unable to apply those rules when she's at Sunday school.

Let's take the example of Sunday school. You do an ecological inventory to see what your kindergarten-age daughter will need to be able to do. You will want to observe ahead of time, and discuss your child's needs with the teacher. Find out what happens during most sessions.

In that setting, she might be told:

Come into the room and hang your jacket on the hook.
Sit down on the blue carpet.
Wait quietly for the teacher to begin.
Watch the teacher.
Don't poke other children.
Listen to the story.
Sing with the other kids.
Don't take more than your share of refreshments.

An older child might need to learn how to go on a bus trip with a club or team:

Make sure you have your backpack with your books and tapes.
Get on the bus and sit down in your seat.
No jumping, screaming, or poking other people.
Talk to the other children.
If you get tired or bored, take out a book and read it.

And so on. Teaching these skills takes more than just stating them once; your child will need practice. But children with Asperger Syndrome generally are likely to be interested in rules, and remember them, so this tendency can be harnessed.

Settings

You can't cover every setting your child is likely to encounter, and teach each setting before it's ever encountered. But you can get a head start on some likely places and circumstances, and prepare your child for the outings that are most likely. Here are some useful starting points:

- the street, apartment building, or neighborhood
- stores where you are likely to take your child

- places with waiting rooms (doctor, dentist, other offices)
- library
- playground
- visits to (and from) family friends
- movies and other amusements
- religious services
- play dates and visits with peers
- public restrooms
- travel, including the airport, the airplane, the train
- farms or rural areas where sensory issues like heat, bugs, and smells might be a concern
- your workplace, if you take your child for a visit

When you take your young child to the store or to the library or to the bank, the two of you are in an ideal setting for learning. Initially, you may be concerned mostly with getting your business completed without any upset from your child. But as she learns to stay composed during outings, and perhaps gets rewarded when she does, you will have a chance to use these times to explain the ways of the world to her.

For example, you can talk to a child about food, or nutrition, or money in elementary terms while you shop. Studies have shown that children with PDDs learn a skill like shopping better when the learning takes place in the store, rather than in a classroom. They are more likely to learn how to respond to the cues found there—the signs that say what each aisle contains, for example, or where the cashiers are. And they are less likely to be upset or confused when they shop on their own.

You can also build support for your child by capitalizing on the tendency of many children with Asperger Syndrome to relate better to adults than to their peers. While this tendency should be counteracted, there are times when it can help ingratiate the child with other adults. For example, one boy who loves books spends a lot of time at the library. His solemn, "professorial" conversations and queries delight the staff and volunteers. His adult friends welcome him, and keep an eye on him when he is at the library on his own.

Skills

Following are some of the particular skills your child can work on. Some will come fairly easily, but others may require considerable time and practice. Some may not be mastered until your child is quite a bit older, but it's good to begin the basics early.

Let's begin with skills appropriate to quite young children—preschoolers and those in the first few years of elementary school. (Some of these, of course, are the same essential skills you taught at very early ages, and that we've discussed in chapter 5.)

- knowing when to be quiet (in church, at a musical performance, or at a solemn occasion)
- using correct tone and volume of voice (at the park or playground, as opposed to a church service)
- understanding rules of proximity (no poking or touching; how far away to stand when talking with someone)
- initiating a conversation
- sharing
- taking turns
- making eye contact and smiling
- using polite phrases and requests
- waiting in line
- knowing boundaries of privacy (what part of a store or another person's house or body is off limits)
- answering the telephone

For older children, the following skills should be addressed:

- making introductions
- making telephone calls
- ordering at a restaurant
- knowing how to behave in a public restroom when the parent is not present (For example, boys need to know how to deal with

urinals differently than they would with their toilet at home.)

· interpreting facial expressions and body language
· understanding figures of speech, particularly those likely to be used by her age group
· responding to authority figures

In addition, there are conversational skills that your child will need to be taught explicitly. Among them:

· Selection of topic, and who is likely to be interested in it. An anecdote about family members will be of more interest to other family members than to a stranger. Your child's detailed discussion of geography may go over better with adults than with other children.

· Ways of shifting topics. This includes recognizing when to change the subject, and being able to recognize and use the phrases that signal a change: "By the way" and "That reminds me" are examples.

· The need to provide background information. This is a challenge for people who have trouble with theory-of-mind tasks, but it is not uncommon in the typical populations as well. Many people will happily tell you all about their relatives and friends, without assessing your familiarity with, or interest in, these people.

· Reading of cues that other people use (smiling, nodding, eye-rolling, watch-checking).

When teaching conversational skills, in particular, remember that your child is likely to remember and understand the idea of rules, and of a "right" way of doing things. When you talk about listening to the other person talk, for example, you can present that as the same kind of rule as sharing, or taking turns. We don't interrupt when other people are talking. We wait for our turn.

You can also harness another trait common among children with Asperger Syndrome: the special area of interest. Your child can come to understand that it's fun to talk with other people about her favorite topic. If she can learn the rules, explain herself well, give others a chance to ask questions, and listen politely to them, she will have more fun sharing her interest with others.

The Issue of Safety

Children with Asperger Syndrome can be frighteningly oblivious to signs of danger, because of their inability to sort out important cues from the environment and act on them quickly.

Your best approach is to supervise your child carefully during these years, continue to teach and remind, and remember that your child is likely to remember and apply rules—including safety rules— more readily than most children.

Crossing the street is a major concern when children leave the house on their own. A child who seems old enough to remember to look both ways may fail to do so because she was distracted by odd noises in traffic, the drone of an airplane, the odors of exhaust. Teach "crossing the street" as a specific skill, and be sure to supervise your child until you are sure she has learned this essential skill. Don't be daunted by other parents who yell at your child or glare at you because your child "should" be able to do this at her age.

You may find yourself supervising your child more than parents of other children the same age. Don't be discouraged from doing what you think is right for your child. There are other safety issues that require judgment, along with rules, and you should be confident that your child can handle them before she goes out on her own. These include the crucial distinction between people she knows and strangers, and the difference between "friendly" strangers (store clerks and police officers, for example), and unfamiliar or unsavory people.

In addition, you will need to teach the concept of "good

touch/bad touch," explicitly, and monitor her understanding of these crucial issues of privacy and safety. You will likely use strategies and concrete content appropriate to your child's age, but will need to develop specific rules, including reporting strategies, specifically for your child.

For example, while you teach your child the appropriate skills for being polite in a social setting—a neighborhood picnic, for example, you will also have to teach her the appropriate behavior if she should be approached by a stranger. Those would include not speaking, running away, yelling, and most important, telling a trusted adult. These are difficult skills indeed, but she will be able to learn and remember them with practice.

Helping Your Child Decode the Hidden Social Agenda

Typical kids are able to learn social rules and apply them to a range of situations. They get the gist, the essentials of a social rule, and with help, are able to generalize it. Not so for children with Asperger Syndrome. Skills and rules learned in one setting won't seem obvious in another setting.

Therefore, your child will have to learn to improve her ability to understand the hidden social agenda that other children pick up readily. And even if she never quite decodes it, she can learn to use other techniques to help her behave appropriately in a range of settings. This is helpful when your child begins school, and the classroom rules and routines can seem overwhelming at first.

Sometimes, a child is in a situation where the rules don't apply (or she's forgotten the rule). I often advise my young patients who are in a group situation and aren't sure how to behave to do what the other kids are doing. Even if it's not exactly the *right* thing, at least several kids will be doing it, and the child with Asperger Syndrome won't stand out as much.

For example, a group of children are at a neighborhood shopping center and a sports celebrity comes and stops to sign autographs for the kids. The event is unpredictable and exciting, and your child is unlikely to have been prepared for it. If your child knows to watch the other kids in such an event, she'll know that the way to behave—to fit in—is likely to gather around, look enthusiastic, and perhaps shake hands with the athlete.

The reason this method is advised is that kids with Asperger Syndrome often turn to adults for cues and advice when they need help. They tend to imitate adult manners, and may have stilted mannerisms. Advising them to model other children does two things: it helps reference them toward the peer group they need to figure out, and over time, it makes it more likely that their behaviors will fit in with those of the group.

A variation that can be used in a group setting, like a classroom, is to observe an older or well-behaved student in a group of children. In classroom situations, I've observed that these students are most likely to exhibit consistently the behaviors that are expected in that setting. If a child really isn't certain whether to sit quietly, or get out her workbook, or push her chair under her desk, she can usually get it by doing what the "model" does.

Ultimately, however, your child's best hope for figuring out a social situation is to develop her *own* critical thinking skills. Children with Asperger Syndrome have great difficulty "thinking out of the box," and often get stuck responding only in one way because they don't know any other way, even if their response doesn't fit the situation.

For example, six-year-old Maria knows that the correct behavior at the playground is to climb on the jungle gym and swing on the swings. At the hardware store with her father, Maria sees a display of play equipment, and begins to climb with enthusiasm (despite the "For Display Only—Keep Off" sign) before she is captured by her father. Maria has forgotten the "store" rule about not touching things, and applied the "playground" rule of climbing and playing freely.

To get your child to "think out of the box," you can expand the "What-if?" lessons we discussed in chapter 5 as your child gets older. Together, you and your child can brainstorm some situations that she is likely to encounter. Here are some "What ifs?" I've worked with. You'll come up with ones that suit your child's situation. For a young child, you might ask: "What if you wanted to play with a toy, and another child had it, and there was only one of that toy?"

Some answers kids suggest: Grab the toy. Ask to use the toy. Ask to use the toy next. Offer another toy in exchange. Punch the kid. Scream. Give up.

For an older child, the question might be, "What if another kid calls you a name?"

Possible answers: Punch the kid. Cry. Do nothing. Call him the same name back. Ask him if he's saying that to be mean, or just playing.

Here are some other "What ifs?" you might consider:

- What if someone you don't know offers to give you a ride in their car?
- What if you are in the library being quiet, but somebody near you is being very loud?
- What if you are out walking Spot and the leash breaks and Spot runs away?
- What if you are in the school auditorium, and you get a stomach ache?
- What if you answer the phone and the caller wants to leave a message for Daddy?

Another useful tool for helping kids learn skills and expectations for social situations is a series of scenarios called Social Stories. They can be adapted to any situation you might find yourself wanting to teach your child. We discuss these more in chapter 8.

My Child: An Owner's Manual

As you and your child build up your repertoire of settings and skills, you might find it useful to keep detailed records of what works and what doesn't work for your child in the settings she encounters. Your child's Owner's Manual could be in the form of a loose-leaf notebook or a file on your computer, which allows you to update it periodically. This will be a good "shorthand" for teachers, baby-sitters, and others to follow in your absence.

For example, write down what rules and skills you've set. Your instructions might be as simple as, "Caitlin dislikes peanut butter but will usually eat any other kind of sandwich. But she becomes upset if the sandwich has been cut in half."

Or, "It's important to follow Benjamin's bedtime routine specifically. After he brushes his teeth and gets in bed, he gets two bedtime stories, and the last one *must* be "Babar." Or, "Before you take Roger into a new setting, be sure to remind him about the proper behavior for each. He needs to remember that at the library he should be quiet, select a book, sit down, and read. But if he goes to a friend's house, remind him that he is expected to greet people, suggest games, and so on." In time, your own child can refer to it for guidance. Make sure you list what worked and what *didn't (or won't)* work. No sense in repeating past mistakes.

Reaching Out for Support

"One thing about having a child with Asperger Syndrome is that it is incredibly isolating," one mother told me. "Not only do you sometimes feel alone with your difficulties, but you also feel that you can't take your child places, because people won't understand the tantrums and outbursts or unusual behavior."

And it's true, of course—children who regularly misbehave in public bring stress to one and all. But as we discussed in chapter 5, a great deal of stress can be reduced by preparation, skill building, and practice. But there's another dimension. The more your neighbors, acquaintances, and community are part of the equation, the less isolated you and your child will feel, and the more support you will find.

If you have been working to help your child build social skills, you are doing part of the job. The other part of your task is getting others to be willing to accept your child's unusual behavior, and give her the benefit of the doubt when things don't go smoothly. You've begun this process in the way you discussed your child's condition with outsiders. As we discussed in chapter 3, you have sized up the empathy level of the people you come in contact with, and handled the issue of disclosure differently for different people.

As you work on helping build community support for your child, you will find the best results come from being open with other adults and children, and getting them on board. An adult who has some understanding of Asperger Syndrome will be less likely to belittle or avoid your child. A child who is sympathetic will be less likely to tease.

"Ben has a social learning disability called Asperger Syndrome," you might tell your child's coach. "He has difficulty learning how to understand social experiences, and we often have to teach him concretely. It's like a foreign language to him; we're teaching him gradually, and he's learning. He'll do his best if you tell him very plainly what to expect and what to do. He actually likes it when people tell him what to do."

One mother finds the most support when she talks about her son's sensory issues. She explains that he gets upset, or withdraws, when he is uncomfortable, and then she explains exactly what things upset him. Most people can relate fairly easily to the idea of being disturbed by loud noises, scratchy clothes, or an overheated room.

"People usually feel compassionate about this, and respond by giving the child a bit more leeway in terms of being different," she says. The same compassion is often evident when parents describe their child's difficulties in terms of anxieties that other people can understand. "Sylvia gets upset easily when unexpected things happen. When she doesn't quite know what to expect, or what's expected of her, it feels sort of like stage fright. She gets nervous."

While your child is quite young, it will be up to you to find activities and groups and settings where she can develop her social skills and a sense of community. It may begin with a walk to the corner deli, and a discussion with the owner, followed by your child's practice lesson in buying a treat.

Another good place to start may be your religious community, where structured programs for children are often well organized and supportive. You can talk with the staff about how to integrate your child into the group, and perhaps how to involve the other children in being supportive of your child's needs, as William's teammates were.

It may be athletics, if that's what you and your child enjoy and if your community's athletic programs have a spirit of inclusiveness. Most community-oriented athletic programs (as opposed to those focused on serious competition) are fairly lenient about including children who may not quite get the gist of team play. But be careful, because some programs are intense and high-pressure at an early age. Such an activity would not likely be a positive experience for your child. Soccer, for example, is a marvelous sport for most children, but is often difficult for children with Asperger Syndrome because it involves quick decisions on the field and interactions with others. And some community leagues are highly competitive.

Or your focus of involvement may be with Asperger Syndrome support groups, both for adults and children. Whatever avenue you use to journey toward a nurturing community experience, you will have better success if you are directly involved in that community—the youth sports teams always need coaches, the churches and synagogues have much work for volunteers, and neighborhoods always welcome involved residents who help out with the block party or the summer picnic.

"We parents of kids with Asperger Syndrome do best if we are the Scout troop leader, or the PTA president, or the volunteer coach," a parent told me. "Then we are involved, and can help our kids along with the group. And also, we are more likely to know what's going on.

Our kids often don't understand everything that's happening, and they often don't tell us what they do know."

You may have to take the same proactive role with your child's play dates. You know, more than the other parents, how important it is to structure the occasion, rather than simply let the kids "go out and play." You may have to host more than your share, but it's important to provide your child with the opportunity to socialize while she and the other children are young and willing to allow their parents to set up social contacts.

During these activities, it's wise to set up activities that your child likes that also appeal to other kids. Computer games are fine, especially the kind that permit two players (otherwise your child may monopolize the game while the guest looks on). Pokémon and other popular activities that involve collecting and trading of character cards are often enjoyable.

If possible (and it may not always be possible) identify and invite sympathetic, confident children who may provide a buffer between your child and other children and be more protective. Clearly, we don't launch our young children out the door on a wing and a prayer. We've got to be there with them. You will invest considerable time and attention at this point in your child's development, so that she can venture safely beyond the family. Over time, however, you will see how much progress she has made, and you'll recognize that there is more and more she can handle on her own.

As she starts school, she will have more opportunities for social and intellectual growth. She will also face new and greater challenges in both of those areas. We'll discuss those opportunities and challenges in the next chapters.

7

The Code

Your Child's School Experience

"Read between the lines," her language arts teacher would say to her as the class discussed a passage. "But there are no words between the lines," Alison would say with a puzzled look.

"Why don't people just tell me what they mean?" she said recently to me in pained frustration. Almost everybody she knew spoke in a secret code. People used words in ways that had hidden meanings that, it seemed, everyone but Alison could understand—everyone, that is, except very young children, although even they seemed to learn the code by the time they were five or six. Maybe that explained why it was easier for her to play with her younger cousins than her older ones.

She recalled having this problem throughout her school years. Like the time she became upset in second grade science and began to cry. Alison remembers that she wasn't allowed to continue to talk about which penguins molt and which do not, because the teacher wanted to continue her lesson about the differences between warm-blooded and cold-blooded animals.

Or the time in algebra, when the teacher reprimanded her

for complaining loudly (and forcefully) about the unfairness of an open-notes quiz. Alison believed that, because the teacher had told everyone to study for the quiz in advance, his sudden decision to allow students to use their notes was breaking the rules and just plain unfair. Her classmates didn't share her view and were not amused.

Alison realized that learning the Code was possible, but it would take more effort than mastering geometry. Memorizing the code seemed the best approach, but that task often required an interpreter. By middle school she learned to ask an adult for a translation, but not before she learned never to ask a middle-school classmate! "There should be a rule book for the Code," she sighed with resignation.

Now, as she was about to graduate from the tenuous security of her high school into the unpredictability of the summer and community college in the fall, she was even more apprehensive. Most people just didn't understand how big a problem this could be. What was worse, she didn't really know how to figure the Code out on her own, whether during lessons in the classroom or in the halls with her peers. The difference in intent of the phrases "Knock it off" and "You knocked my socks off!" eluded her. While the social risks of her misperceptions were considerable, frequently she was unaware of them.

Alison's struggles with school are typical of children with Asperger Syndrome. Like Alison, your child may learn certain material seemingly without effort, but "the Code"—the hidden social curriculum—may make it difficult for him to succeed. Other children with Asperger Syndrome find school challenging for other reasons: sensory overload, chaotic or unpredictable classroom settings, or social isolation and rejection.

For many children the early grades go fairly well, as they acquire basic facts and do clearly explained, straightforward school projects. But as they move through the grades, more and more work requires a mastery of complex relationships. Literature and novels become more subtle and mystifying.

Your child will need special support to manage his school experience. Fortunately, we've learned a great deal about how to teach and support children with Asperger Syndrome in classroom settings. First, let's examine what support your child is entitled to under the law, and then we'll look at what a good and effective program for your child should look like.

What the Law Guarantees Your Child with Asperger Syndrome

Since 1994, when Asperger Syndrome became an official diagnostic category, it has been much easier for parents to obtain the educational services and support that their children require. Under Public Law 94–142, passed originally in 1975, and reauthorized as the Individuals with Disabilities Education Act (IDEA), Congress guarantees "a free appropriate public education" for all children with disabilities.

This means that your child is entitled to an appropriate education, tailored toward his needs, within "the least restrictive environment." This means that your child should be educated in an environment that is as close as possible to that in which all children are educated—meaning, in most cases, the regular classroom.

The law provides protections for children who are denied appropriate services, and for parents who are not satisfied with their child's placement or degree of support. Parents have the right to be involved in decisions made about their child, and to challenge and appeal decisions they feel are not appropriate.

It's important to remember that the federal law provides a minimum level of service that all states must guarantee for their children. Some states have chosen to provide more guarantees, and a higher level of service. Your child has a legal right to the basic rights provided by the federal law, along with additional rights and services provided by your state.

Even if a student with Asperger Syndrome does not require an Individual Education Program (IEP), he may benefit from, and be eligible for, assistance under Section 504 of the Rehabilitation Act of 1973. These services, commonly called a Section 504 Plan, are developed with your school system and provide instructional assistance in school. A 504 Plan can be particularly helpful to a student moving from a special education placement to a regular education placement.

For information on your state's policies toward special education, and the services available to children with Asperger Syndrome, contact your local school district or the state education agency (see the Resources section).

Chances are, your child will receive his education in a variety of settings. They may include a traditional classroom with one teacher and children with a range of abilities. They may include a special education "resource room," where children with Asperger Syndrome (and possibly other disabilities) go for certain classes and services. There may be an "inclusion" class, a team-taught classroom in which both regular education and special education students learn together from a team of teachers. Services may also include sessions with a range of specialists, from physical or occupational therapists to language or reading specialists and school counselors.

The law says that children must be educated in the least restrictive environment, which means that they should be with other, typical children where that is appropriate. This does not mean that providing children with support in special classrooms is restrictive. It may be the best way for a child with Asperger Syndrome to be able to concentrate and learn.

Educating children with disabilities alongside their nondisabled peers is called integration, or "mainstreaming," and it is a fundamental goal in placement. However, integration has both supporters and detractors when it's applied to children with Asperger Syndrome. That's because the disability itself is so linked to issues of peer interaction, self-esteem, and difficulties in group and crowded settings.

Those with concerns about mainstreaming point out that students with Asperger Syndrome are often overwhelmed by the sensory, transition, and social challenges of a regular classroom. They may be incapable of focusing or learning in a typical classroom. Thus, that setting may not be "least restrictive," nor necessarily "appropriate," because the child's learning is impeded.

Ultimately, the way a child's brain works should drive not only what he is taught, but where he is taught. If your child suffers greatly from distress and anxiety in large groups, and is unable to get much benefit from regular classroom experience, it may be necessary to give him alternate settings for many of his activities. However, keep in mind that how well a child does in a classroom depends on how much support he receives there, and how effective that support is. This decision should be made by you *and* his teachers, and other professionals who know him well. But remember: *your* participation is key.

How to Make Sure Those Services Are Provided

Depending on the age at which your child was diagnosed, you may already have worked with your school on getting special services and support. In fact, the federal law guarantees children certain services from infancy, if they are deemed "at risk" of developmental delays. However, as we've pointed out, most children with Asperger Syndrome don't exhibit unusual deficits that young. It's only as they approach school age, or are in school, that a clear idea of their diagnosis may emerge.

Thus, you may find yourself entering the special education world as your child enters kindergarten or elementary school. The key document in special education services is your child's IEP. Under the law, your child is entitled to an educational program that takes into account his particular needs. No two children have precisely the same needs, whatever their diagnosis. So the IEP is the keystone of what, and how, your child will receive services.

The IEP process usually begins when either the parents or a teacher requests an evaluation. Parents give permission for the child to be tested and evaluated, and one or more meetings are scheduled to discuss what services are best for the child. The IEP document is prepared by the school's Child Study Team or Planning and Placement Team, and must include full parental participation.

The IEP should include the following:

- your child's present level of development, based on testing or other evaluation
- your child's developmental strengths and needs
- the specific educational services your child will receive
- standards for determining whether the goals of the IEP are being met
- the extent to which your child will participate in regular education programs
- any other interventions or services your child may need
- parent concerns, if they wish to add to the report

Your IEP meetings, and what you contribute to your child's IEP, are the core of your advocacy for your child. This is your opportunity to explain what you think will or will not work with your child, what he needs, and what goals you think are realistic.

The tone of these meetings can range from totally supportive and collegial on one end of the spectrum, to dismissive and bureaucratic on the other. Some parents find IEP meetings wonderfully helpful and positive, while for others they are a trial. Here are some suggestions to get your IEP meetings off to a good start:

- Bring a spouse, partner, or advocate to the meeting.
- Know your rights.
- Know your child; specifically, know what works and what doesn't.
- Be cooperative and assertive. That means you should expect coop-

eration, but be prepared to assert your rights if your child's needs aren't being addressed.

- Know about Asperger Syndrome and speak up about what you know will help and what will not help your child.
- Take detailed notes during the meeting. Or tape record the meeting; just make sure everyone at the meeting knows it is being taped.
- When you receive an official copy of the IEP, compare it with your notes and return it with corrections if necessary.

The quality and appropriateness of services vary greatly according to where you live. Some families have great difficulty getting school bureaucracies to approve or provide services for their children. If this is your experience, remember that you have the law on your side. The law provides for a grievance procedure, including mediation and an impartial "due process" hearing, if you dispute the school's placement or services. However, if you are dissatisfied, it's usually best to begin by trying to resolve the dispute informally and resorting to the more formal grievance process only as needed.

Classroom Settings That Support Your Child

My colleagues at Yale University's Child Study Center, psychologist Ami Klin and child psychiatrist Fred Volkmar, have described the particular settings in which children with Asperger Syndrome are likely to do their best, and the strategies that are likely to help them. Their book, *Asperger Syndrome,* edited by Klin, Volkmar, and Sparrow (Guilford Press, 2000), outlines much of this material, and we are grateful for their permission to share some of their insights.

The setting should be small. Children with Asperger Syndrome require considerable individual attention. Small work groups and the opportunity to break tasks down into very small steps help them learn. Although children may do some of their work in a standard-size classroom, those areas where they need particular interventions are better kept small.

The environment should be orderly and predictable. As we've seen, children with Asperger Syndrome do best in settings that are predictable, in which they feel they know what to expect. Transitions should be minimized where possible. Of course, a typical school day does involve lots of transitions from one activity to another. Children are asked to put away their social studies books and prepare for a math lesson. One day, the students have music after lunch; the next day, it's gym.

It's wise to minimize transitions where possible, and prepare for them when they're necessary. The teacher should explain them in advance, give visual cues and verbal reminders, and help the child rehearse the change. Thus, the teacher can remind your child that today is Tuesday, and he will go directly to the music room after lunch. He can be reminded again before lunch, and a lunchroom aide can help make sure he gets where he is supposed to go.

It's important to maintain a consistent daily routine as much as possible. When changes in the routine will occur, again, the teacher should provide ample warning. A predictable setting and routine are not only comforting and stabilizing for children with Asperger Syndrome, but they can provide a "home base" for gradually increasing their ability to tolerate change. The more comfortable your child is with his setting and routine, the more he'll feel able to adjust to surprises and changes in routine. Learning to tolerate transitions is a gradual process, but kids do improve with practice.

Other classroom arrangements that seem to help involve minimizing distraction. Fairly uncluttered classrooms and bulletin boards are more likely to help a child with Asperger Syndrome focus on what's important and be able to ignore secondary cues.

Seating arrangements matter, too. It's often best if your child is seated toward the front of the classroom, and away from peers who either annoy him, or whose behavior isn't a good model for the social learning he so much needs.

Real-life settings are best for teaching socialization. Thus, lunchroom behavior is best learned in the lunchroom, hallway behavior in the hallway, and so on for playground, classroom, music room, and other school settings. Naturally, this means the entire staff—gym teachers, lunchroom aides, and so on—must be briefed on how to work with your child and promote acceptable behavior and social skills in these settings. This, incidentally, is one reason why educating your child in a setting along with typical children, where possible, is usually the best way to enhance your child's social development, because that setting provides models of the kind of typical social skills he will need to learn.

Teaching Strategies That Help Your Child Succeed

The most important points to keep in mind when planning or evaluating an educational program for a student with Asperger Syndrome are:

Individualize. The program will have to be carefully designed to meet the needs of your child, with your child's pattern of strengths and weaknesses. Children with Asperger Syndrome vary widely in what they need in an academic setting; one size does not fit all.

Coordinate. Educational services will be provided to your child by a team, including the classroom teacher and specialists who may include a reading specialist, language specialist, occupational therapist, and others, along with the physical education teacher, librarian, and even lunchroom aides and bus drivers. Those who provide services to your child should coordinate their efforts so everyone is on the same page. The team should have a clearly designated case manager or "point person."

Be consistent. Children with Asperger Syndrome yearn for consistency and predictability. Consistency is their best friend. It's essential that everyone who works with your child be aware of his needs, and that they use—within reason—the same techniques to teach him.

Remember that Asperger Syndrome is a social learning disability. The teacher should keep this utmost in mind and seize opportunities for social learning in the classroom. The teacher also needs to remember that the social dynamic may affect how a child performs. So a child who performs well in small, organized groups may have difficulty in a busy classroom; a child who knows the material may have trouble demonstrating that mastery if he is distracted or upset by what other children in the classroom are doing.

Emphasize rote instruction. The best technique for teaching basic content is in rote fashion, stating facts and repeating them. Children with Asperger Syndrome need to have the material laid plainly before them.

Ironically, for several generations, education has been moving away from drill, memorization, and rote instruction toward more creative and flexible approaches: stories, role-playing, creative projects, and other techniques that help typical students put material into context. Children with Asperger Syndrome, however, often do better in a more old-fashioned setting in which the teacher presents information, and the child learns and applies it.

Avoid ambiguity. Just as Alison had difficulty with certain phrases, your child will also be baffled by figurative use of language. His teacher should either avoid them, or carefully explain what they mean. Here are some examples:

- Idiom: "He jumped the gun." "Don't have a cow." "That begs the question."
- Sarcasm: "Oh, that was thoughtful of you" (to a child who is being inconsiderate).
- Jokes: Most depend on double meanings, which must be explained.

· Nicknames: These confuse kids with Asperger Syndrome because they appear to mock or make fun of a person, but actually are intended to be friendly. Similarly, names like "Pal" or "Son" used informally can confuse kids.

Teachers can learn techniques for signaling to the child with Asperger Syndrome whether they are being literal, or exaggerating, or making a joke. An unobtrusive sign, or simply saying, "Of course I'm joking now," can help the child understand how to process the information.

Use part-to-whole sequences. Students with Asperger Syndrome learn complex material best if they are able to use inductive, rather than deductive, reasoning. This is a crucial distinction, because many students learn better using a combination of both inductive and deductive reasoning.

With inductive reasoning, you start with the specific, and move outward toward generalities. You learn about Earth, then the solar system, then the stars and galaxies.

Deductive reasoning begins with the broad concept, and from that broad explanation, specific information can be deduced. For example, a biology unit on reproduction might begin with a broad look at the necessity for living organisms to propagate themselves and then break the issue down into plant and animal kingdoms, sexual and asexual reproduction, and so on.

A child with Asperger Syndrome does better when each piece of the information is explained first, and the connections to larger concepts are added later. It's best to give the child a clear, explicit example, then gradually add more examples, before tying a concept together in broader terms.

For example, a unit on the life cycle of butterflies might use pictures and descriptions of a caterpillar, a chrysalis, an emerging butterfly, and a butterfly laying eggs to show each piece of the process called metamorphosis. The child will understand metamorphosis better if the parts of the concept are emphasized at first, and tied together later.

Recognize that a good memory can be deceptive. "Memorization" or "intellectualized learning" should not be misunderstood as conceptual learning, unless the skills are firmly demonstrated. Students with Asperger Syndrome may memorize to excess but lack the fundamental understanding of a concept. The teacher should be sure to investigate how deeply the child understands the subject.

Strengths and Weaknesses in Students with Asperger Syndrome

As we have seen, students with Asperger Syndrome often have impressive academic strengths. These may include reading (the decoding part, but not necessarily the comprehension part), mathematics, general memorization of facts, and logical thinking. They often are highly skilled with computers. These strengths should be acknowledged and harnessed in the classroom wherever possible.

Children with Asperger Syndrome often have "splinter skills," or areas of considerable ability. Often, these relate to the child's particular interest, or may include skills such as memorization. Enrichment activities are appropriate for a child with Asperger Syndrome who shows great proficiency in an area, although enrichment should be provided with an understanding of the deficits that sometimes come with those talents. Thus, if your child's expertise in volcanoes consistently brings him prizes in the science fair, he should certainly be given enrichment opportunities such as trips to the natural science museum. But if his interest is so obsessive that it crowds out other areas, that needs to be balanced with opportunities to pursue other activities.

Often, however, students with Asperger Syndrome have learning disabilities, sometimes in the areas of written expression, mathematics, or reading comprehension, along with difficulties with personal organization. Thus, it's a good idea to enlist the services of the reading specialist in the early assessment process, from first grade forward, to ensure that a child's decoding skills do not mask more complex reading comprehension difficulties.

The child's IEP should identify any specific learning disabilities and outline a plan for addressing them. In addition, children with Asperger Syndrome often have motor difficulties that affect a range of skills from athletic ability to handwriting. If related services are needed such as occupational or physical therapy, these should be developed from a functional approach, rather than only a theoretical approach, meaning that they should focus on specific tasks that the child needs help with, such as handwriting, tolerating different foods or sounds, or adjusting to crowded places.

Students with Asperger Syndrome often have trouble organizing their writing, and may have trouble completing tests on time. When this is the case, it's appropriate for the teacher to adapt assignments and allow for more time for testing.

In addition, children should be taught to use the impressive computer resources that are available to help students write, organize projects, and plan and organize their activities. (See the Resources section.) Basic word processing techniques are essential, especially for students who have trouble with handwriting. They should include keyboarding, creating documents, using spelling and grammar checking programs, and so on.

Here are some other areas of difficulty for students with Asperger Syndrome, and some strategies for dealing with them:

Communication. It's important to engage the child with Asperger Syndrome in conversation within the classroom, even though that may be difficult for him. Materials can be arranged in such a way that the child needs to ask for information, or request help. For example, rather than just handing a book to the child, the teacher can say, "When you're ready for the encyclopedia, please come and ask me." Other friendly students can be enlisted to serve as helpers to the child with Asperger Syndrome in order to develop functional language skills.

Problems of social communication include difficulty shifting topics, ending a conversation, expanding a topic, discussing a topic of interest to others (but not oneself), and so on. Strategies for teaching these social and communication skills should be taught specifically. We'll discuss more about specific social strategies in chapter 8.

It is essential to have a communication specialist involved who understands pragmatic language development and social skills training. This specialist can work with everyone who interacts with your child so that everyone is attuned to opportunities to help your child develop communication skills.

Unusual interests. Students with Asperger Syndrome have many areas of unusual or eccentric interests, and while these sometimes interfere with their participation and performance, they can also be used productively.

Designate a "time and place for eccentricities." One child, for example, was only permitted to ask questions about his favorite topic, snakes, during recess. His teachers, and some cooperative children, made themselves available during recess and learned immense amounts of information about snakes, but once the bell rang the discussion ended.

When a child manages to stop himself independently, in a sense self-regulating his obsession, he should be praised and rewarded. Similarly, time to enjoy the favorite interest can be offered as the reward for completing a task that the child is not interested in.

It's appropriate to individualize assignments and special projects to coincide with highly developed interest areas. Book reports or long-term science assignments on such topics of interest are helpful. Teaching a student to read and research *beyond* his area of interest is important, too.

Mentoring is a helpful strategy, whereby a student's area of interest is linked to an adult with a similar interest. That way, the interest becomes a source of pride and accomplishment, and it provides an opportunity for social interaction. Many adults with Asperger Syndrome look back on a mentor as a key individual in their development and learning.

Organization and concentration. Beyond specific learning disabilities, an overall problem with organization is almost universal. Although some children with Asperger Syndrome appear to be very orderly when it comes to organizing their collections or demanding that their shoes be kept in a certain arrangement, nearly all have trouble with the more global aspects associated with executive function.

This reveals itself in a whole host of school-related problems such as:

· forgotten assignments
· confusion about how to begin a project
· difficulty organizing thoughts into an essay or project
· lost papers and books
· notes to parents that never arrive home

There are numerous ways to help kids organize themselves better, and they range from simple checklists, to visual prompts, to computer programs that help kids organize their work. For example, a simple picture of a pencil, taped to the front of the child's notebook, may help remind him to bring his pencil to class next time.

He'll be able to do a better job organizing his material for a term paper if each component of the paper is represented by a picture, or a written item on a checklist, and these prompts are presented in sequence as they are discussed.

For example, a paper on the Anasazi Indians might include sections on the land where they lived, how they built their houses, their arts and crafts, and why we think their civilization disappeared. Each section could be illustrated—with a map, a cliff dwelling, a pot, and a question mark. These prompts would give the child a sequence to follow as he writes.

Communication between school and home should never depend on the child, although the child should be encouraged to take notes home. The school should never assume that they arrive, however, and should have a clear system of communicating with parents. E-mail is a very helpful method for regular communication between parents and teachers.

Timed work sessions are often difficult for a student, but where they are unavoidable it is often important to identify a visual end point. For example, the class may be given a worksheet of fifty arithmetic problems, but your child is expected to complete only ten because the task will take him longer. Something as simple as drawing a line after the tenth problem signifies a closure point for him, and enables him to concentrate better on the task.

Sometimes, the way information is presented in class can make it difficult for your child. Students with Asperger Syndrome have a hard time shifting their attention—for example, from the teacher to the material on the board or the screen of the overhead projector. It's difficult for them to process visual and auditory information at the same time. Students will need to learn to improve their abilities to integrate visual and verbal information simultaneously. But this process takes time, and in the meantime, they need material presented clearly in a way they can handle.

The teacher should assume that a child has difficulty organizing material, even if he appears to have mastered the content. Graphic organizers, study guides, outlines, key word summaries or key concept summaries all help organize and highlight what's important.

In dealing with problems of organization it is also important to teach independence. Early in your child's educational career, the focus will be on close supervision and "hyperorganization." Gradually, the instructional strategies should offer more flexibility and independence to the student. When your child works independently, when he monitors and controls his own behavior successfully, he should be reinforced, praised, and rewarded.

Sensory issues. Discuss with your child's classroom teacher the kinds of stimuli that your child finds upsetting, and see if together you can work on ways to minimize them. Your child can be seated away from a humming water cooler or be positioned so that the sun's glare doesn't distract him. He might be excused the rotating task of cleaning the hamster's cage if he's oversensitive to smells.

In addition, decide on an acceptable way for your child to calm himself and mask upsetting stimuli. Are there settings or activities in which it's acceptable for him to listen to soothing music on a Walkman? Might he quietly fiddle with worry beads or a paper clip, or fold origami? It's best if you and the teacher—with your child's input—have discussed reasonable accommodations ahead of time.

Trouble with novelty and change. As we know, it's difficult for children with Asperger Syndrome to cope with novelty and unanticipated change. These things are unavoidable in a school setting, however, so your child's program should include methods of teaching strategies for dealing with change. You can reinforce these strategies at home, using the "Oops" and "What-if?" techniques we've described, and the Social Stories discussed in the next chapter.

However, it's particularly helpful for your child to be able to work on these issues at school. Learning that takes place in the relevant context is more likely to be retained and applied appropriately. Your child can rehearse a strategy for dealing with lunchroom problems in a small setting and then practice in an empty lunchroom, and then apply the knowledge during an actual lunch period. Adults can introduce novelty and change into the routine gradually, allowing your child to practice these skills in manageable doses.

A particular ritual might signal the opening and closing of an activity—something as simple as taking out materials or putting materials away. Your teacher and child can work together to establish specific routines for the nonacademic areas of the school day, such as moving between classes in the hallway, lunch, assemblies, and so on.

When things don't go well, it's important for the teacher to use mistakes as teaching opportunities. Frequently occurring troublesome situations should be dealt with immediately, without the assumption that the child will ultimately learn from experience. The technique of performing "Social Autopsies" of situations that went wrong, in order to learn from them, is discussed in chapter 8.

The Social Dimension of Learning

Jonathan is a whiz at mathematics, and excels at logic questions. He stands at the board and solves complex problems that have stumped his classmates. But put him in a group, and set him to a task of working as part of a team, and he invariably ends up lashing out in anger. He alternates between insisting that everything be done his way, and bursting into tears because the others "aren't being fair." He has great difficulty with the give-and-take that is part of the learning experience that group projects offer.

A classroom is more than an interaction between the teacher and the child, or the child and the material and the concepts. The other children in the classroom have an enormous impact on the quality of every child's learning experience. A typical child will be more successful in a setting in which he feels accepted, liked, and inspired by his classmates; he will do less well when he feels frightened, disliked, or bored by the other children.

This is true for a child with Asperger Syndrome, as well. However, your child will have more trouble interacting socially and feeling accepted than typical children. Similarly, he will have more difficulty learning from his peers and benefiting from group projects and team experiences. He'll also have trouble generalizing skills that he's learned at home, or in small group settings, to the classroom.

More difficulty, yes, but peers offer great benefits, as well as great hurdles, for the child with Asperger Syndrome. Let's examine ways that teachers can support your child's social learning and help harness peer interactions to help your child academically.

A No-Teasing Zone

First, the teacher must explain and enforce a "zero tolerance policy" for verbal abuse, including subtle verbal "slams." This policy has to be explained to the entire class and firmly enforced. It's always a good idea to raise the consciousness of all students about diversity and differences. Students who transgress should be dealt with clearly, so the child with Asperger Syndrome understands that it's not OK for others to victimize him.

Just as importantly, the child must learn that *his* words can be hurtful, too. He might tease others, and interpret the giggling and attention he receives from classmates as support. "Class clowns" develop in this way. Concrete feedback on what is OK to say and what is not will help. For example, "Jokes about people's bodies are not OK because they make people feel bad."

Playing to His Strengths

Your child will have greater success in school if he has skills that can be used to attract positive attention and social bids. These "social magnet skills" might include an expertise in dinosaurs in the early grades, or an ability with math or computers or chess later on. For example, in kindergarten, precocious readers are viewed as higher-status students by their classmates. If your child is able to read proficiently, or spell, or do multiplication facts, the teacher can engineer a setting in which other children look to that child as an "academic star," and initiate social bids to him to access his information or assistance. Later on, the student with an incredible facility for numbers and orderliness might be a valued member of the Math Olympiad Team.

Buddies, Buffers, and Mentors

An effective strategy for students with Asperger Syndrome is the development of a buddy system, or circles of peers, in which selected students who are sympathetic and also relatively popular help as partners and mentors. The teacher can approach these children and ask if they would be willing to serve as valuable helpers to the child with Asperger Syndrome, praising them for their maturity and sensitivity. Obviously, no child should be forced into service.

These children can serve as layers of insulation around the child with Asperger Syndrome. This provides a group of peers who understand the child, his abilities, and his idiosyncrasies. Beginning this process as early as possible allows for those circles to expand by the addition of new children over time.

For students like Jonathan, the math whiz, it's often helpful to assign group projects with at least one buddy or mentor. This child can remind him to stay on task, and can ease the stress that causes Jonathan's outbursts.

Sometimes the peer support comes from other students with Asperger Syndrome. The school may set up therapeutic experiences in school such as social counseling groups, "lunch bunch" gatherings, or social language groups. These groups can also provide the support that comes only from others who are in the same boat (not necessarily Asperger Syndrome). Moreover, getting to know other children with Asperger Syndrome (whether at school or in other support group settings) can be a great help, and provide your child with a good foundation for reaching out to support groups in later life.

Social Stories are an excellent tool for teaching children with Asperger Syndrome how to handle a particular situation. These short, specific scenarios teach solutions to social experiences by providing clear instructions on how to respond to, and how to interpret, a social challenge. We go into more detail in chapter 8.

Children with Asperger Syndrome can be reminded about the strategy we discussed in chapter 6: Look to their peers when they are unclear about what to do in a certain situation, or how to behave. A three-step classroom strategy might include:

1. Look to your neighbor and do what he is doing.
2. Ask your neighbor what to do and follow his instruction.
3. Raise your hand and ask an adult.

Although your child may eventually end up asking an adult, at least this approach gets him to think in terms of learning behavior from people his own age. Over time, this will reduce the areas in which a child with Asperger Syndrome stands out as different, or odd, in comparison to other children.

Behavior Management

Jonathan behaves well in the classroom, as a rule. The parts of the school day that are most difficult for him are lunch, recess, and gym class. In those settings, he no longer has the familiarity of his room, his regular seat, and a highly structured routine. Instead of finishing his lunch in the cafeteria, for example, he begins to roam the room, singing loudly, swinging his arms, and approaching other children in annoying ways; he walks up to them and falls against them, or into their laps, until they yell at him and push him away. When the lunchroom aide asks why he does this, he says he doesn't know—the other kids don't like him, and he's "stupid."

While Jonathan has suffered from teasing, his real problem in the lunchroom is lack of structure. He does better when he's assigned a seat, when he sits with a buddy at least during part of the session.

It is important for everyone working with your child to understand that what appears to be misbehavior is often due to your child's disability. If he has trouble with anxiety and stress, if he panics in unfamiliar situations, if he misunderstands other children's intent, he is more likely to behave inappropriately. It's possible to minimize outbursts by making sure the child's environment is predictable and consistent, and making sure that he understands the situation and what to do in it.

Your child's teachers can teach strategies for managing stress, such as a voluntary, or personal, "time-out." This allows the child to voluntarily take himself out of play when he feels the need. There should be a safe haven to which he can retreat. He also can learn to anticipate and prepare for challenging experiences (such as going into a crowded auditorium) by wearing a Walkman with his favorite music to screen out noises and to help him remain calm.

When your child does misbehave, it's best to begin not by assuming the behavior is caused by malice or mischief. Better to see if there's been a breakdown in the implementation of a strategy: Has his setting remained predictable? Have his routines been changed? Have adults behaved inconsistently? Only after checking do we assume that the child with Asperger Syndrome has failed to conduct himself properly.

For example, if a child is sent from the classroom for disruptive behavior, it is worth checking to see if something went wrong with his routine. Perhaps on that day there was a substitute teacher who hadn't been briefed on the procedures the child relied on. Misunderstandings on both the child's and teacher's parts can create confusion and compound problems.

Updating Your Child's "Owner's Manual" for the Classroom

If you began building your child's "Owner's Manual" when he was younger, you have a basis for what you and his teachers can construct and update together. Of course, it's an informal document, but much of its insights have probably been incorporated into your child's IEP, which will guide the more official aspects of his education experience.

But it's still worth updating and discussing the manual with your child's teacher. If there are "hot button" topics or "trigger areas" that elicit anxiety, overarousal, or social confusion, these should be identified and addressed. The manual can offer specific solutions for difficult settings, a working paper of survival strategies that are effective.

Like the formal IEP, it should be reviewed with your child, his teachers, and other school personnel who work with him. It should be updated over time, and should include any accommodations and adaptations that your child is permitted.

Ultimately, careful records like the Owner's Manual will become a useful support for your child outside of school as well. It can help others who may assist or work with him. If he goes to college, it can help set forth his strengths and weaknesses as he works with support staff there. And it can help him as an adult, as he advocates for himself and seeks appropriate services on his own.

Bear in mind that your child's formal IEP applies only to his education through high school. But the insights contained in the IEP, along with the Owner's Manual, can help you and your child develop an appropriate program in college.

Let's take another look at Ethan, whom we first met in chapter 2. His story shows how children can thrive when their school environment is nurturing and wise.

Here's how Ethan's parents report on his progress:

> Now in public kindergarten, Ethan is getting extraordinary help. Seven school system professionals work with him several hours a week, providing group-based social skills instruction, anxiety management, sensory and motor planning therapy, and speech and language instruction. Because our town's school system is so excellent, most of these interventions began before Ethan got an actual diagnosis. They were provided separately to deal with the social and physical deficits we saw and the teachers and administrators saw as remediable.
>
> We have noted improvements already in his motor skills and in his ability to initiate a conversation with another child. Our anxiety and dread have lessened. We feel we have come full circle and easily recall the days we marveled at the early signs of intelligence and the idiosyncrasies we still found more endearing than worrisome. We find ourselves, again, much more awed and appreciative of our child's uniqueness.

We've discussed ways to make your child's school experience successful, and ways to help him learn and cope with the school day. Your child has a right to an appropriate education and the support he needs, but it's important to remember that teachers need all the help they can get, too. Remember, your child's teacher is responsible for a large number of children, each with unique abilities and needs. And even though your child's teacher may be well prepared for working with children with Asperger Syndrome, most teachers will also welcome all the input you can provide on how best to work with your child.

The following is a summary of what children with Asperger Syndrome need in the classroom setting, and what strategies help them learn and succeed. It covers some of the approaches we've discussed in this chapter, along with more specific insights tailored for teachers. We're grateful to Karen Williams, of the University of Michigan Medical Center Child and Adolescent Psychiatric Hospital School, for permission to adapt her article.

You may wish to copy the guide and give it to your teacher or show this section of the book to him or her. In either case, it's important to remember that no guide can describe every child; it's your task to explain to the teacher your child's unique personality and interests, and what you think will work and what won't work for your own child.

A SPECIAL MESSAGE TO
MY CHILD'S TEACHER

As you know, my child has been diagnosed with Asperger Syndrome, a developmental disorder that affects his ability to understand and participate normally in social interactions. This affects many aspects of his school experience. There is much about school that is difficult for my child, but I also recognize that having a child with Asperger Syndrome in the classroom presents a challenge to the teacher as well.

The following brief guide is designed to help you understand my child, and to make it easier for you to help him academically, and develop his confidence and social skills.

Children diagnosed with Asperger Syndrome present a special challenge in the school setting. They're often considered eccentric and peculiar by classmates, and their awkward social skills often cause them to become victims of teasing and scapegoating. Clumsiness and an obsessive interest in obscure subjects add to their "odd" demeanor.

Children with Asperger Syndrome have trouble understanding human relationships and the rules of social convention. They may seem naive and lacking in common sense. Their inflexibility and inability to cope with change make them easily stressed and emotionally vulnerable. Most children with Asperger Syndrome are average to above-average in intelligence and have superior rote memories. Their single-minded pursuit of their interests can lead to great achievements later in life.

Asperger Syndrome is considered a disorder at the higher end of the autistic continuum, but people with this disorder are quite different from what we often think of as autistic. One expert described the difference this way: the low-functioning child with autism "lives in a world of his own," whereas the higher-functioning child with autism "lives in our world but in his own way."

Naturally, not all children with Asperger Syndrome are alike. Just as each child has his own unique personality, symptoms vary among these children as well. As a result, there is no exact recipe for classroom approaches that can be provided for every youngster with Asperger Syndrome, just as no one educational method fits the needs of typical children.

Following are descriptions of seven characteristics of Asperger Syndrome, followed by suggestions and classroom strategies for addressing these symptoms. Of course, the suggestions should be tailored to the individual child.

1. INSISTENCE ON SAMENESS

Children with Asperger Syndrome are easily overwhelmed by change, even slight changes. They are highly sensitive to environmental influences, and sometimes engage in rituals. They are anxious and tend to worry obsessively when they do not know what to expect; stress, fatigue, and sensory overload easily throw them off balance.

Programming Suggestions

· Provide a predictable and safe environment. In elementary school classrooms, the child with Asperger Syndrome benefits from knowing where to sit, where to find materials, where to look for information on the blackboard and bulletin board.

· Minimize transitions. Some are unavoidable during the school day, but the more stable the routine, the better for the child with Asperger Syndrome.

· Offer consistent daily routine. It may help to take the child aside at the beginning of the day and outline the day's schedule. Post the day's events on the blackboard or bulletin board, or provide him with a written copy. When the child with Asperger Syndrome understands each day's routine and knows what to expect, he'll be much more able to concentrate on his school work.

· Avoid surprises. Prepare him thoroughly and in advance for special activities, altered schedules, or any other change in routine, regardless of how minimal. If a special guest will come to give a presentation, prepare the child with Asperger Syndrome well in advance, and let him know what to expect. If you will be absent from the class, alert the substitute or another staff member to talk to the child with Asperger Syndrome about the change.

· Inform the child beforehand of any new activity, teacher, or class. Try to expose him to the new situation—an introduction to a new teacher, a visit to a new classroom—as soon as possible after informing him, to keep him from worrying obsessively. For instance, when the child must change schools, he should meet the new teacher, tour the new school, and be told about his new routine well in advance. School assignments from the old school might be provided for the first few days, so that the routine is familiar, even though the environment is new. The new teacher might find out the child's special areas of interest and have related books or activities available on the first day.

2. IMPAIRMENT IN SOCIAL INTERACTION

A child with Asperger Syndrome shows an inability to understand complex rules of social interaction. He may exhibit some or all of the following attributes:

· is naive; seems unaware of "the ways of the world"
· is extremely egocentric; focuses on his own needs and concerns and seems unaware of those of others
· may not like physical contact; may perceive friendly or accidental contact as hostile
· talks "at" people instead of to them
· does not understand jokes, irony, or metaphors
· uses a monotone or stilted, unnatural tone of voice
· uses inappropriate gaze and body language; may stare off to one side instead of at the other person's face in conversation
· is insensitive and lacks tact; may make inappropriate or hurtful comments without realizing that they are offensive
· misinterprets social cues; doesn't understand facial expression and body language (for example, when another person rolls his eyes, backs away in discomfort, or picks up a book to signal the end of a conversation)

- cannot judge "social distance"; may stand too close or otherwise violate the "personal space" of others
- exhibits poor ability to initiate and sustain conversation
- has well-developed speech but poor communication
- is sometimes described as a "little professor" because speaking style is so adultlike and pedantic
- is easily taken advantage of (does not understand that others sometimes lie or trick people)
- usually has a desire to be part of the social world and have friends

Programming Suggestions

- Protect the child from bullying and teasing.

- In the higher age groups, attempt to educate the other children in the classroom about the child with Asperger Syndrome by describing his social problems as a true disability. Even in younger grades, his difficulties can be explained in ways that the children can understand. Explain that everyone has trouble with some things; some kids wear glasses to help them see better, some have asthma and use an inhaler to help them breathe better. A child with Asperger Syndrome has trouble understanding social behavior and needs other people to explain things. Praise classmates when they treat the child with compassion.

- Emphasize to the class the ways in which the child with Asperger Syndrome is especially capable. Create cooperative projects in which the children work together in teams toward a shared goal. The child might be the designated research person who easily finds facts in the encyclopedia, or who reminds others in the group if they have forgotten a step in how the project should be done. In this way, the child's reading skills, vocabulary, memory, and so forth will be viewed as an asset by the other students and help him become more accepted by his peers.

· Most children with Asperger Syndrome want friends but simply don't know how to interact. They should be taught how to react to social cues and be given repertoires of responses to use in various social situations. Teach him what to say and how to say it. For example, you could teach a primary grade student to say, "Did you see (a particular television program) last night?" Model two-way interactions and let him role-play; perhaps you could practice a script for joining a game at recess; some of the time, he could be the child joining, and some of the time, you (or another child) could take that role. For an older child, you could practice conversations about his vacation, or yours. His social judgment will improve if he is taught rules that others pick up intuitively.

· Although your student with Asperger Syndrome may lack personal understanding of the emotions of others, he can learn the correct way to respond. When he's been unintentionally insulting, tactless, or insensitive, he needs a clear explanation of why his behavior was inappropriate and what would have been correct. He needs to learn social skills intellectually. You might say, "John, you told Eric he looks like a pig. That made him feel bad, so he got angry at you. Don't make comments about the way people's bodies look."

· Older students with Asperger Syndrome might benefit from a "buddy system." You can educate one or more sensitive classmates about the situation of the child with Asperger Syndrome and seat them next to each other in the classroom and for other activities. The classmate could look out for the child on the bus, during recess, in the hallways, or in other settings, and attempt to include him in school activities.

· Children with Asperger Syndrome tend to be reclusive, or at least reluctant or unable to initiate social interactions. Encourage active socialization by asking him questions and drawing him into discussions. Limit the time he spends in isolated pursuit of interests. For instance, a teacher's aide seated at the lunch table could actively encourage the child with Asperger Syndrome to participate in a group conversation, not only by asking him questions, but also by subtly reinforcing other children who do the same: The aide might say, "Erica, I'm glad you asked Robert to describe the boat trip he took on his vacation. We enjoyed hearing about that."

3. RESTRICTED RANGE OF INTERESTS

Children with Asperger Syndrome have eccentric preoccupations or odd, intense fixations (sometimes obsessively collecting unusual things). They tend to relentlessly "lecture" on areas of interest, ask repetitive questions about interests, and have trouble letting go of ideas. They often follow their own inclinations regardless of external demands, and sometimes refuse to learn about anything outside their limited field of interest. While this can certainly make it difficult to teach the child, these interests can be used to guide his learning.

Programming Suggestions

· The child with Asperger Syndrome may go to extremes discussing or asking endless questions about isolated interests. It's important to limit this behavior by designating a specific time during the day when the child can talk about a favorite subject. For example, one child who was fixated on animals had innumerable questions about a class pet turtle. The teacher explained to him that he could ask all the questions about the turtle that he wanted to, but only at recess. She made a point to be available to him during recess for these discussions about turtles. This was part of the child's daily routine, and he quickly learned to stop himself when he began asking these questions at other times of the day.

·   Positive reinforcement is helpful. In the case of a relentless question-asker, the teacher might consistently praise him as soon as he pauses and congratulate him for allowing others to speak. He should also be praised for simple, expected social behavior that is taken for granted in other children.

·   Some children with Asperger Syndrome will resist doing assignments outside their area of interest. It's important to be clear that you expect him to complete his classwork, as all children must. Make it clear that he must follow specific rules. At the same time, however, meet him halfway by giving him opportunities to pursue his own interests.

·   For some particularly inflexible children, it may be necessary, at least at first, to individualize all assignments around their interest area. Thus, if the interest is dinosaurs, the teacher might offer grammar sentences, math word problems, and reading and spelling tasks about dinosaurs. Other topics could be introduced gradually into assignments.

·   Students can be given assignments that link their interest to the subject being studied. For example, during a social studies unit about a specific country, a child obsessed with trains might be assigned to research the modes of transportation used by people in that country.

·   Use the child's fixation as a way to broaden his repertoire of interests. For instance, during a unit on rain forests, the student who was obsessed with turtles was encouraged to study not only the animals that lived there, but also the forest itself, as this was the animals' home. He then became interested in learning about the local people who were forced to chop down the animals' forest habitat in order to survive.

4. POOR CONCENTRATION

Children with Asperger Syndrome are often off task and distracted by internal stimuli or sensory issues (such as a rattling air conditioner or uncomfortable clothing). They can be very disorganized and have difficulty sustaining focus on classroom activities. There is a lot going on in a typical classroom, and the child with Asperger Syndrome may have a hard time figuring out what is important and what is not. He may focus on a ladybug crawling on the ceiling, or the sound of the classroom aquarium pump, rather than the teacher's voice. He may tend to withdraw into his own inner world in a manner much more intense than typical daydreaming.

Programming Suggestions

·   Seat the child with Asperger Syndrome at the front of the class and direct frequent questions to him to help him pay attention.

·   He needs a great deal of regimented external structure to be productive in the classroom. You will need to break assignments down into small units, and offer frequent feedback and redirection.

·   Children with severe concentration problems benefit from timed work sessions. This helps them organize themselves. Classwork that is not completed within the time limit (or that is done carelessly within the time limit) must be made up during the child's own time (during recess, for example, or during the time used for pursuit of special interests). This can motivate him to focus and get the work done within a reasonable time.

·   Children with Asperger Syndrome can sometimes be stubborn. Firm expectations and a structured program teach them that obeying the rules brings rewards. This kind of program motivates the child to be productive. If he sees himself as competent, it builds his self-esteem and lowers his stress levels.

· Poor concentration, slow writing speed, and severe disorganization may make it necessary to lessen the child's homework and classwork load. He may benefit from time in a resource room where a special education teacher can provide the additional structure he needs to complete classwork and homework. Some children with Asperger Syndrome are so unable to concentrate that homework can be unproductive and highly stressful, both for the child and for his parents.

· Work out a nonverbal signal with the child (such as a gentle pat on the shoulder) for times when he is not paying attention.

· If a buddy system is used, seat the child's buddy next to him so the buddy can remind him to return to task or listen to the lesson.

· Actively encourage the child to leave his thoughts behind and refocus on the real world.

· For young children, even free play needs to be structured, because they can become immersed in solitary, ritualized fantasy play. Establish specific activities that the child can pursue during free play; while the other children select an activity on their own, the child with Asperger Syndrome could have a specific book selected or activity planned.

· Encourage a child with Asperger Syndrome to play a board game with one or two others under close supervision. This not only structures play, but offers an opportunity to practice social skills.

5. POOR MOTOR COORDINATION

Children with Asperger Syndrome often are physically clumsy and awkward. They may have stiff, awkward gaits and have a hard time playing games involving motor skills. They also often have fine motor deficits that can cause penmanship problems, and make it hard for them to take notes and draw pictures.

Programming Suggestions

· Refer the child with Asperger Syndrome for an adaptive physical education program if gross motor problems interfere significantly with his participation.

· Involve the child in a health/fitness curriculum in physical education, rather than in a competitive sports program.

· Do not push the child to participate in competitive sports if he finds it frustrating. Most children with Asperger Syndrome lack the social understanding involved in coordinating one's own actions with those of others on a team. Bear in mind, however, that some children enjoy team sports if other team members are supportive.

· Children with Asperger Syndrome may require a highly individualized program to help them with handwriting. It might involve tracing and copying on paper, along with motor patterning on the blackboard. The teacher guides the child's hand repeatedly through the formation of letters and letter connections and also uses a verbal script that describes how to make the letter. Once the child commits the script to memory, he can talk himself through the letter formations independently.

·   Younger children benefit from guidelines drawn on paper that help them control the size and uniformity of the letters they write. This also forces them to take the time to write carefully.

·   When assigning timed units of work, make sure the child's slower writing speed is taken into account.

·   The child may need more time than his peers to complete exams. Taking exams in the resource room not only offers more time but would also provide the added structure and teacher redirection the child needs to focus on the task at hand.

·   Pursue evaluation and treatment by an occupational therapist if fine motor difficulties interfere significantly with letter formation, writing, or daily living skills such as buttoning clothing, and so forth.

6. ACADEMIC DIFFICULTIES

Children with Asperger Syndrome usually have average to above-average intelligence (especially in the verbal area), but lack high-level thinking and comprehension skills. They tend to be very literal: Their images are concrete, and abstraction is poor. Their pedantic speaking style and impressive vocabularies give the impression that they understand what they are talking about, when in reality they may be merely parroting what they have heard or read. The child frequently has an excellent rote memory, but it is mechanical in nature; he may respond like a video that plays in set sequence. Problem-solving skills are poor.

Programming Suggestions

·   Learning should be rewarding and not anxiety-provoking. Design the child's projects and assignments so that he experiences success. For example, in a unit on the American Revolution, when other students are asked to write essays on the complex events preceding the Boston Tea Party, this child might contribute by making a map of Boston Harbor, showing where the key events took place.

· Offer added explanation and try to simplify when lesson concepts are abstract. If you are discussing the Middle East and mention that camels were described as "Ships of the Desert," that metaphor may be easily understood by most of the class. For your student with Asperger Syndrome, you would need to explain the camel's significance in moving people and cargo across the terrain.

· Capitalize on the child's exceptional memory; retaining factual information may well be one of his great strengths.

· The child with Asperger Syndrome will have a hard time understanding emotional nuances, multiple levels of meaning, and relationship issues as presented in novels. Either explain them explicitly, or adapt his assignments to focus on other aspects of the book.

· The child may write in a repetitious manner, flitting from one subject to the next, sometimes with incorrect word connotations. He may not know the difference between general knowledge and personal ideas and therefore assume the teacher will understand his sometimes abstruse expressions.

· Children with Asperger Syndrome often have excellent reading recognition skills, but weak language comprehension. Do not assume they understand what they so fluently read.

7. EMOTIONAL VULNERABILITY

Children with Asperger Syndrome have the intelligence to compete in regular education, but they often do not have the emotional resources to cope with the demands of the classroom. They are easily stressed. They often have low self-esteem, and they are often very self-critical and unable to tolerate making mistakes. Adolescents may be prone to depression. Rage reactions and temper outbursts are common in response to stress and frustration. They rarely seem relaxed and are easily overwhelmed when things are not as their rigid views dictate they should be. Interacting with people and coping with the ordinary demands of everyday life take continual Herculean effort.

Programming Suggestions

· Prevent outbursts by offering a high level of consistency. To lower stress, prepare the child for changes in daily routine. He is likely to become fearful, angry, and upset in the face of forced or unexpected changes.

· Teach the child how to cope when stress overwhelms him, to prevent outbursts. Help the child write a list of very concrete steps that can be followed when he becomes upset. For example: "One: Breathe deeply three times; Two: Count the fingers on your right hand slowly three times; Three: Ask to see the special education teacher"; and so on. Include a ritualized behavior that the child finds comforting on the list. Write these steps on a card that he can keep in his pocket so that they are readily available; sometimes just the knowledge that he has the list of helpful tips will reduce his anxiety level.

· When speaking to a student with Asperger Syndrome, be aware that he won't be able to understand the emotional content of speech the way most students do. For example, a tone of sympathy, or disappointment, or sarcasm will be hard for the student to discern. Be calm, predictable, and matter-of-fact in interactions with the child, while clearly indicating compassion and patience. Hans Asperger, the physician for whom this syndrome is named, remarked that "the teacher who does not understand that it is necessary to teach children seemingly obvious things will feel impatient and irritated."

·   Do not expect the child with Asperger Syndrome to acknowledge that he or she is sad or depressed. In the same way that he can't perceive the feelings of others, he can also be unaware of his own feelings. He may often cover up his depression and deny its symptoms.

·   Teachers must be alert to changes in behavior that may indicate depression. These may include even greater levels of disorganization, inattentiveness, and isolation; decreased stress threshold; chronic fatigue; crying; suicidal remarks; and so on. Do not accept the child's assessment in these cases that he is "OK."

·   Report symptoms to the child's therapist or make a mental health referral so that he can be evaluated for depression and receive treatment if this is needed. Because these children are often unable to assess their own emotions and cannot seek comfort from others, it is critical that depression be diagnosed quickly.

·   Be aware that adolescents with Asperger Syndrome are especially prone to depression. Social skills are highly valued in adolescence and the student realizes he is different and has difficulty forming normal relationships. Academic work often becomes more abstract, and the student finds assignments more difficult and complex. But symptoms of depression or unhappiness are not always obvious. In one case, teachers noted that a student was no longer crying over math assignments and therefore believed that he was coping much better. In reality, he had been escaping further into his inner world in order to avoid math, and that caused his decreased organization and productivity.

· It is critical that adolescents with Asperger Syndrome who are mainstreamed have an identified support staff member with whom they can check in at least once daily. This person can assess how well the student is coping by meeting with him daily and gathering observations from other teachers.

· Children must receive academic assistance as soon as difficulties in a particular area are noted. These children are quickly overwhelmed and react much more severely to failure than do other children.

· Children who are very fragile emotionally may need placement in a highly structured special education classroom that can offer an individualized academic program. These children require a learning environment in which they see themselves as competent and productive. Accordingly, keeping them in the mainstream, where they cannot grasp concepts or complete assignments, serves only to lower their self-concept, increase their withdrawal, and set the stage for a depressive disorder. In some situations, a personal aide can be assigned to the child, rather than special education placement. The aide can offer emotional support, structure, and consistent feedback.

Teachers can play a vital role in helping children with Asperger Syndrome learn to negotiate the world around them. Because these children are frequently unable to express their fears and anxieties, it is up to the adults in their lives to make it worthwhile for them to leave their safe inner fantasy lives for the uncertainties of the external world.

Professionals who work with these youngsters in schools must provide the external structure, organization, and stability that they lack. Using creative teaching strategies with individuals who have Asperger Syndrome is critical, not only to help them succeed academically, but also to help them feel less alienated from other human beings and less overwhelmed by the ordinary demands of everyday life.

8

The Medieval Women's Clothing Club

Communication and Social Issues in Childhood

Paula's first science project in third grade had been about moths and butterflies. Her teacher liked it so much that Paula thought her classmates would like it too, so at recess she dedicated herself to finding good examples on the playground to share with other children. They were less amused after the first week, uninterested by the second, and starting to avoid her by the third.

This just didn't make sense to her, but a lot of things like this just didn't make sense. Wouldn't you think that everyone who made such a fuss about her insects for the project would certainly want to learn more? It was so hard to understand what other people really wanted or were thinking about sometimes. She wanted to have friends, but wanting them was a lot easier than figuring out how to make them.

Recently, her teacher had suggested that students in class develop "recess clubs" for sharing interests or activities with other students. Because the insects had not been a successful social draw, Paula decided on another area of interest.

For some time, Paula had been fascinated by the clothing worn by women in medieval England. Royalty, courtiers, and commoners all had prescribed styles, ranging from purely decorative to entirely functional. She had already committed to memory the timeline of the medieval era, the major historical events, and the dates of birth, ascension, and death of the kings and queens of the period. The evolution of their clothing styles was just another exciting aspect of her continuing discovery. Paula had noticed that some of the girls in her class enjoyed talking about things they were wearing to school, and so she decided with a now typical resolve to start the Medieval Women's Clothing Club.

She decided that invitations were the best way to offer her soon-to-be new friends a place in her club, so the design became a special project. With her dogged determination, she spent hours on the computer, locating pictures of clothing styles along with the dates they were in fashion. With more searching she found pictures of men's clothing, too (that would interest boys in joining her club). Neatly tracing and coloring the pictures, she prepared a set of invitations for school.

At the end of morning work on a Monday in February, Paula asked her teacher if she could talk about her "recess club" to the class. With self-confidence and certainty, Paula handed out the invitations, hoping she had enough for all who would be interested.

Unfortunately, Paula's recess club was not the success she'd hoped for. The Medieval Women's Clothing Club was able to attract some nibbles; a few girls, drawn to the intriguing drawings of dresses, congregated around Paula. But it soon became evident that another purpose of the club was to give Paula a forum for listing everything she knew about the Middle Ages, and that was plenty.

One of the major distinctions between autism and Asperger

Syndrome is that children with autism quite frequently show little or no interest in peer interaction, while children with Asperger Syndrome often seek companionship. The difficulty for these children, as we see in Paula's situation, is that they are often unable to make friends in the intuitive way that most children do.

In this chapter, we'll look at the central issue in Asperger Syndrome: the social and communication disability at its heart, how that affects the lives of children and their families, and how these deficits can be counteracted with strategies that have been shown to help.

"My Wonderful Child Has No Friends"

One of the sorrows of parents of children with Asperger Syndrome is that their children, quite wonderful children, are often without close friends. This is a painful process for the children themselves, although it may not be as intense in the early elementary years as it may be later and in adolescence, when "fitting in" is crucial, and the awareness that one is not fitting in can be a source of great frustration.

But it's devastating for parents, too. Most of us want to know that our children will be appreciated by others, and will be able to forge attachments with their peers. It's much more fundamental than a concern about social status, or that our child be "popular." We want our children to find friendship, and the fulfillment it brings, just as we hope our children will be intelligent and healthy and good.

It can be a great sorrow for parents to watch other children sailing through their social lives with such apparent ease. In fact, other parents may complain about their children's hectic social lives, and recount how the house is always filled with children, the slamming of doors, the ringing of the telephone, the endless parties and car pools. As the parent of a child with Asperger Syndrome who may be quite isolated socially, you find yourself wishing you had their "problems."

It's particularly painful for parent and child when the child with Asperger Syndrome is teased. In this sense, the condition is particularly cruel, since the oddities of behavior draw attention from other children, and the inability to figure out social subtleties leaves the child vulnerable to the unkindness of others.

However, as we have discussed in chapter 6, the picture is not as bleak as it may seem. But in order to be able to help your child, you will need to appreciate the particular difficulties your child faces socially and work with her on her skills.

Why Children with Asperger Syndrome Don't "Fit In"

The child with Asperger Syndrome may appear odd or annoying to other children in several ways.

Verbal skills. As we have discussed, children with Asperger Syndrome may have unusual tonal qualities in their spoken voices, including either sing-song or flat intonation. In addition, they often speak in a stilted or unnatural way, and in a way that strikes other children as overly formal or adult.

In addition, like Alison, they have difficulty with the conversational give-and-take that's part of play. Kids use a whole range of idiomatic phrases, and the child who "doesn't get it" stands out. For example, the phrase "Oh, really?" delivered with dripping sarcasm, sounds perilously close to "Really!" spoken with astonishment after someone's clever remark.

One child had heard a friend use the phrase, "Don't sweat the small stuff." An adult who wanted to check his comprehension asked if he knew what it meant. "Sure," he replied. "It's when you use the smallest exercise equipment and it doesn't make you sweat like on the big equipment."

Children usually sense that they don't follow what's going on, and may think they are being teased when they are actually being included. Dane, a sixth grader, was with two acquaintances who were having great fun creating nicknames for each other. In their efforts to include him, they called him "Danish." He became hurt and offended, and ran away from a social encounter that was actually friendly and positive.

Odd behavior. Children with Asperger Syndrome may exhibit unusual movements and postures, or engage in repeated movements that make them stand out. In addition, they may have behaviors that are inherently irritating to others, such as screaming, hitting, poking, and grabbing at others, or bursting into tears. Often these behaviors—usually the sign of anxiety—occur without warning.

Unusual appearance. Children with Asperger Syndrome, while usually quite normal in general appearance, often stand out because of unusual dress or hairstyle. Sometimes this is because their clothing and hairstyles are not up-to-date, and sometimes it's because they cling to comfortable clothing and resist aspects of grooming that they find uncomfortable.

Sam, for example, stands out because he almost never gets a haircut. Going to the barber or hairstylist upsets him, so he keeps this shaggy unkempt hairdo. Chad tends to wear old T-shirts and sweatshirts with outdated images on them (one, from his early childhood, has Sylvester the Cat on it).

Motor deficits. Physical awkwardness may range from poor athletic skills to difficulty manipulating small items such as a pair of scissors or cosmetic or hair grooming implements, to difficulty playing a musical instrument.

Apparent rudeness or inappropriate statements. Children with Asperger Syndrome are unlikely to know when to keep their observations to themselves, and may offend others unintentionally.

Inflexibility. Children with Asperger Syndrome have a tendency to dislike change and innovation and play, and to hold firm convictions. Just as it is more difficult for them to learn turn-taking as small children, it is difficult for them to master the concept that "not everyone can be right all the time," or that it is acceptable to "agree to disagree."

A tendency to dominate play. During social interactions, a child with Asperger Syndrome may tolerate social contact only as long as the other children play the game by her rules. She may be unwilling or unable to join in games or imaginative scenarios suggested or generated by others, in part because someone else's game will require that she be flexible and deal with the unexpected. As Tony Attwood points out, "to include other children is to risk an alternative script, interpretation, or conclusion—that is, you have to share and cope with different ideas."

Other children, even those who mean well, may be baffled by this behavior. They understand tantrums, for example, but not those that often come out of the blue. They understand being "bossy" when the bossy child incurs an advantage, but they are puzzled when a child insists loudly that none of the twelve-year-olds at the restaurant table (including herself) should be allowed to order from the under-twelve children's menu.

Often, younger children are relatively content to do without the company of others, but as the years pass, they are more likely to sense their own isolation and wish for friendship. This desire becomes more intense as adolescence begins. Unfortunately, if the early isolation ensured that the fundamental social skills were not learned, the task of forging friendships in adolescence will be difficult indeed.

Children with Asperger Syndrome may seek out adults for companionship, rather than their age-mates, because usually adults are more tolerant of children's social inadequacies and may be more likely to be impressed by—or at least tolerant of—the child's favorite topics of conversation. That is why, throughout this book, I've emphasized the importance of working to build social skills.

How to Help Your Child Enhance Social Skills

In earlier chapters, we addressed some of the social and behavioral skills appropriate to younger children. Now that your child is in school and interacting with other school-age children, it's important to consider what she should master at this stage in her life.

By her early elementary years, your child will—ideally—have gained some control over behaviors that cause her difficulties in public (tantrums, unusual fidgeting, or repetitive behavior). She presumably will have learned to greet people, and to engage in some elements of play, including turn-taking.

During the years of middle childhood, she will strive toward mastery of more mature skills, although, naturally, not all children will progress smoothly toward these goals.

The task is two-fold. Your child must be herself—she is not required to "stop" having Asperger Syndrome, or to abandon her fascination with windmills or penguins, but she must also build her skills in order to increase her opportunities for a fulfilling, independent life. Therefore, it is important to help your child increase her links with her peers, her opportunities for social learning, and her ability to blend in with the crowd to the extent that this is possible. At the same time, it is important to reach out and seek supportive environments, where your child's idiosyncrasies will be, to some extent, accepted.

If this task seems daunting, remember that you have been working with your child since her early childhood to build these skills, and you and she have come a long way. What you will be doing now is expanding the groundwork laid in earlier years. Just as she learned the "rule" about saying "please" at age four, now that she is eight, she will be able to learn the "rule" about looking another child in the eye and saying, "Hi. I'm in fourth grade. What grade are you in?"

For children who have been diagnosed only recently, it's important not to dwell on the fact that you may not have known to teach these things specifically when your child was younger. What's important is to concentrate on the present, and teach her the skills she needs now and in the future.

Teaching social skills involves several steps. The specific skill or behavior itself needs to be identified. (Earlier, I described an ecological inventory as one means of identifying these skills; other examples are listed below.) Next, a time and place for initial instruction must be determined. Starting with a small setting, perhaps one-to-one, often helps. The other teaching strategies described earlier—breaking a skill down into small steps, teaching from part-to-whole, staying concrete and avoiding abstract or nonliteral interpretations and concepts—all are applicable here.

Finally, once the skills have been mastered in a smaller situation, they must be expanded—generalized—to lots of real-world experiences. Sometimes simple practice in new places is all that it takes. Other times, a cue card or a reminder will help the child remember strategies and behavior in new situations.

But, as we've seen, learning the rules isn't enough. Life is too complex and too changeable for us to master its mysteries with a simple rule book. We need to be able to adjust to new situations and to unexpected turns of events. That's what's so difficult for kids with Asperger Syndrome. One boy, who had learned in his school Pragmatics group to use the phrase, "Have a nice day," had to be taught all over that it sounds peculiar when said at eight o'clock at night.

Here are some of the social skills that are appropriate to the elementary school years.

· Monitoring and displaying emotion. This includes smiling and nodding appropriately, and recognizing facial expressions in others that suggest mood. You can ask your child to practice with you as you stand side-by-side before a mirror. You can display a happy smile, a frown, a polite nod, and so forth, and ask her to identify and then imitate your expression.

· Understanding basic social rules, such as speaking politely to adults, not pushing in line, asking for food politely. This might include responding appropriately to conversational attempts by others. (Question: "How was your vacation?" Simple response: "It was great. We went to Cape Cod.")

· Learning to write down some attributes of a child she has just met—favorite television programs, family members, pets, and so on. She can review this list privately before visiting that child, so they have some conversational openings at hand. Of course, the list needs to be updated so it doesn't become outdated.

· Knowing some appropriate leisure skills, other than the particular specialized interest. These might include listening to music, swimming, or hiking.

· Behaving appropriately in small group settings, such as after-school clubs or small social gatherings.

· Limiting obsessive rule-enforcing and accepting that one doesn't have to be right all the time. It's helpful for children to practice phrases that can be used instead of outbursts. ("You may be right" or "I see your point, but . . .")

It's important to remember that children with Asperger Syndrome develop social behaviors around interests first, then relationships. This means that a child is more likely to forge a relationship if both children are interested in the same thing, than if the other child is pleasant or appealing for some other reason.

Seven-year-old Stephanie, for example, has an intense interest in horses. She collects pictures of horses, draws horses, studies all the breeds of horses, and is looking forward to her first riding lesson. When Stephanie's parents arrange a play date for her and a friend, it will be much more successful if the other child shares an interest in horses. This shared interest will overshadow other traits that typical children focus on (whether the other child is "nice" or not).

The kinds of activities that are likely to lead to companionship and opportunities to develop social skills, therefore, are those that involve an interest that the child already possesses, and that the others in the group share. It might be Astronomy Club at school, or getting together with other kids for computer games.

Social Stories

Carol Gray, an educational consultant who works with children with PDDs, has developed a powerful technique for helping children with Asperger Syndrome get a clear picture of social situations they may encounter. In her books, *Social Stories* and *The New Social Stories,* she presents dozens of simple outlines that break down everyday situations into plain steps and sequences.

Take walking down the hall at school, for example. Typical kids usually figure out how to get around the school building without problems during the first few days; they learn the rules about running, about which hallways lead where, about how to wait in line outside the cafeteria. They may violate the rules from time to time, but it's not because they don't understand them.

But children with Asperger Syndrome don't learn this automatically. Not only are they at risk for violating rules they have trouble understanding, but they also often feel a heightened sense of anxiety about open-ended situations.

Social Stories are helpful on several fronts. They help a child prepare for a new situation, they help a child review a situation that has caused trouble before, and they help the child alleviate anxiety about a stressful situation.

Here's an example of a Social Story, titled "Going Places at School." The story was written to help a student who stood too close, ran, or bumped kids in line. Note how precise and explicit the story is.

At school, we do not sit at our desks all day long. We go to a number of other places, both inside and outside of the building.

Some of the places we go are: to Specials, to the cafeteria, out for recess, and to and from our buses.

Most of the time, when we go from place to place in school, the students are in a line.

Students in line stand pretty close to each other.

When I am getting in line, it is important not to run into other students.

When I am standing in line, it is important to be careful so that I do not bump, hit, or poke other students.

When I am in places such as the classroom, the hallway, or at recess, it is important to be careful so that I do not bump, hit, or poke other students.

If I run into other students, or bump, hit, or poke them, they will not be safe, and neither will I.

Someone could get hurt.

Also, if I run into other students, or bump, hit, or poke them, my classmates might get upset with me because I am not being careful and considerate.

Being careful and considerate when I go from place to place with my classmates is a safe way to behave.

My classmates, my teachers, and my parents will be happy that I am acting in such a responsible way.

For an older child who is volunteering at the animal shelter, a Social Story might go as follows:

I like working with animals, and being around other people who like animals, too.

When I go into the shelter, I smile and say hello to the other volunteers.

I put my jacket in the office.

I check the bulletin board for my schedule.

I write down my duties for the day. I do this so I won't forget and become upset.

I go visit the dogs and see if they have enough food.

I go to the office and wait behind the desk. I can read, if no one comes in.

I also play with the cats if no one comes in.

When people come into the office, I greet them and ask if I can help them.

If I don't know the answer to a question, I ask Mrs. Barnes.

When I work hard and do a good job, my boss will know I'm a good volunteer. I'll be happy, too, because I can keep working with animals.

The idea is simple indeed, and you as a parent can apply it in many situations in your child's social and home life. You can generate Social Stories for an upcoming family gathering, or a play date that's been arranged with another child. You can also use Social Stories to correct a problem that has occurred.

Thus, if your child became upset and hit another child because the other child teased her (or she believed she had been teased), you could develop a Social Story that gives her a way to behave, including asking if the other child was indeed teasing.

For example, she might be taught to check:

When someone teases me, first I look around to see if other kids are being teased in the same way. (This helps a child separate real teasing from well-intentioned silliness.)

If it's just me, I ask the kid who is teasing, "Are you teasing me?" (Sometimes this question stops a teaser in his tracks. This at least gives a well-intentioned child the opportunity to explain that his statement was just in fun and not intended unkindly.)

If the other child is teasing, I can just ignore it.

An essential element of Social Stories is the balance of the types of sentences that make up the statements. Carol Gray suggests several types:

Descriptive: We stand in line.

Perspective: We do this so people don't get hurt.

Directive: I keep my hands to myself.

Control: It's important to remember not to bump or hit.

It's important to balance the types of sentences, so that those that tell the child what to do (directive and control) are balanced by sentences that explain and provide context (descriptive and perspective). Indeed, for children with Asperger Syndrome, the perspective and descriptive sentences are of great importance.

Other tools for helping children with their social skills include Social Scripts (which you or your child's teacher can make up), which clearly lay out the words one might use in a particular situation.

If your family is going on a vacation, you could practice how your child might have a casual conversation with another child on a train. Your script could be as follows:

"Hi. My name is Samantha. What's your name?"

After the other child's response, your child could say, "I live in San Francisco. Where do you live?"

You can move on to friendly questions about favorite television programs, where your vacation destination is, and so on.

Of course, these scripts must be taught and practiced with the understanding that sometimes people respond in a way that isn't predictable. Here's where your efforts to teach flexibility come into play. Once a script has been mastered, for example, you can introduce some unusual variations. "What if you turn to the other child and say, 'Hello, what's your name?' and the other child answers in a foreign language?" "What if the person asks a question you can't answer?" Come up with possible scenarios, but underscore that surprises in social interaction are part of life, and your child will survive them.

Gray has also developed Comic Strip Conversations to help teach children more developed conversational skills. Using stick figures and thought balloons, this technique allows children to visualize rules of conversation that are quite hard to explain. This approach is quite useful in helping children work on avoiding typical conversational errors that include:

· interrupting
· tossing in irrelevant details
· non sequiturs—failure to use transition phrases
· failure to add enough background
· failure to assess the other person's need for more information
· stating an opinion in an argumentative way

Comic Strip Conversations help lay out the more subtle aspects of conversation in a visual way, and permit you and your child to practice areas that give her particular trouble.

Another technique, developed by Richard LaVoie, is called Social Autopsies. As you can imagine, they're used when an event or a social encounter did not go well. They're conducted as investigations, *not punishments*. After a problematic social encounter, the child meets with a teacher or parent and talks over what happened, what the result was (whether someone was hurt, or offended, for example). Then they develop a plan to try to ensure that the mistake doesn't happen again.

For example, suppose your child has behaved badly on the school bus. A Social Autopsy might be handled as follows, either in a question-answer format, or with a worksheet.

> **What happened?**
> *I wanted James to make room for me to sit next to him and he wouldn't move his backpack, so I threw the backpack on the floor and then James yelled at me so I pushed him off the seat so I could sit down.*
> **What was the social error?**
> *Throwing James's backpack and pushing him.*

Who was hurt by the social error?

James, because people don't like to be pushed, and me, because he got mad at me and I got in trouble.

What should be done to correct the error?

I can apologize to James and the bus driver.

What could be done next time?

I ask James to make room, and if he doesn't, I could find another place to sit.

Social Stories, Social Scripts, and Social Autopsies all have the same characteristic: They are ways of teaching children with Asperger Syndrome how to understand the social world, behave better, prepare themselves for new situations, and learn from their errors. You can apply the principles informally any time, as you talk with your child about the day's schedule, or evaluate an awkward social moment and discuss how to do better next time.

Social Conversation

While students with Asperger Syndrome often have a lot to say, their manner of conversation may be a problem for listeners. Social conversation skills should be taught explicitly. Psychologists Ronald Leaf and John McEachin have developed an excellent skill sequence for this, published in their book *Work in Progress* (DRL Press, New York, 1998). It includes such skills as:

maintaining appropriate distance (not too close, not too far)
maintaining appropriate body language (for example, no excessive
    slouching, grimacing, sprawling, or hopping)
maintaining appropriate eye contact when talking with a peer
maintaining appropriate eye contact when talking in groups
refraining from inappropriate touching
acknowledging statements of the other person (nod, smile, and so on)

refraining from interrupting or cutting off

listening to what the other person says

staying on topic (no abrupt shifts of topic or jumping around)

bringing up a new topic gracefully

leaving old topics behind when the conversation has changed topics

staying attuned to what the other person finds interesting

allowing others to have turns to talk

refraining from talking over the other person

ending the conversation gracefully

maintaining appropriate volume

These skills should be taught, and practiced, as one would with other social skills. As always, practice and positive performance feedback are essential.

How to Structure a Supportive Social Environment

It's clear by now that your child's development, and the strategies you will use to help her, grow by building on what has been learned earlier. Thus, the skills your very young child learned in your home became the basis of the more sophisticated skills she has learned in her neighborhood or preschool.

Now, as a school-age child, she is at the stage in life when friendship is becoming important. The following activities, selected with care and with attention to her abilities and interests, can provide valuable socialization and learning.

Athletics. For many children with Asperger Syndrome, individual sports may be a better choice than team sports. This concept of "personal best"—in a sense, competing against oneself instead of another team—is helpful in athletics and in school, too. It allows the child to develop gradually, and de-emphasizes competition. Activities such as horseback riding, swimming, running, or ice skating build esteem, pride, physical strength, and coordination. And individual sports can provide social benefits even without the benefit of a team, since people often congregate to play them, and they provide excellent openings for conversation.

Team sports may be inappropriate for some children with Asperger Syndrome because it's often very difficult for them to keep up with the complexities and pressures of soccer, basketball, or baseball. However, there certainly are exceptions—William, in chapter 6, derived great benefit from team sports, and we'll see below what can happen when the adults and the other kids are supportive.

Computer games. Although these can certainly become an obsession, they do provide the child with Asperger Syndrome with an activity that other children are eager to share. This is especially true with two-player systems, where both can play together. Plus, computer skills are often a "splinter skill," and an area where they can feel confident and competent.

Scouts and hobby clubs. Groups that emphasize chess, collecting, computers, or other hobbies can bring children together around an interest or area of competence as long as they are well structured.

How Other Children Can Help a Child with Asperger Syndrome, and Vice Versa

The following story was told by a group of typical children who were puzzled by the behavior of a classmate with an autism spectrum disorder, but eager to reach out to him as well. What they came up with might provide a useful starting place for discussions you have with relatives and friends, with teachers and coaches, and with interested children who might be sympathetic supporters of your child with a little help.

"Kris was walking around outside by himself, and we thought he was lonely. He would just kick the ball around by himself. We wanted Kris to play with us, but he wouldn't play our games. He liked balls and stuff, so we gave him a ball and he just kicked it real high. We decided that if somebody could catch it, they'd score one point. Lots of other kids would come over to play, like ten or fifteen kids, and that's how the whole thing started."

So began the evolution of Krisball, a game played by kicking the ball high into the air, to be caught by someone. As the designated kicker, Kris always had an integral role; the game simply couldn't be played without him. For the other kids, it was a reminder of the hidden talents of a child with a disability; for Kris, it was a source of participation, social learning, and pride.

Eventually, those same kids and several others came up with the following tips for other children who know someone with Asperger Syndrome or other disabilities (originally published by my son, Evan, and I in *Autism and Asperger Digest*).

Tips for Being a Friend with a Student with Asperger Syndrome

· Treat them like anyone else, and talk to them like you would talk to another one of your friends. Don't be too formal, and don't talk to them like they're a little kid.

· Don't tease kids with Asperger Syndrome. Sometimes they don't understand the teasing, or sometimes they think that you're being friendly when you're really not. If other kids tease them, pull the other kid aside and tell him to stop.

· Explain to other kids that weird behavior isn't the fault of the child with Asperger Syndrome; it's just how they are.

· Don't ignore them, even if you think they don't notice you.

· Find out about their disability. Read some stuff on the Internet or ask a teacher or a guidance counselor for books. You could also ask their mom or dad when you see them.

·   Ask a teacher or guidance counselor if you're confused about something the kid is doing. There's a reason why they do things. Try to figure it out so you can help them better.

·   Don't get mad at them for something they do that bothers you, or something they don't do that they should. Kids with Asperger Syndrome just can't help it sometimes.

·   Be patient because sometimes it takes kids with Asperger Syndrome longer to do something, or to answer a question.

·   Take time to say "hi" whenever you see them. Even when you're in a hurry and pass them in the hall, just say "hi."

·   Instead of saying, "I don't want to be friendly with him because he has special needs," just try to get to know him.

·   Don't be afraid to go up to them if they need help.

·   Just work with them and try to help them learn. That will make you feel good, and will help them, too.

·   Encourage them to try new things because sometimes they're afraid to try new stuff.

·   If they have a special ability or interest, try to find ways to let them use it. That way other people will think of them as smart.

·   Say something to them when they do good things. You can cheer, give high-fives, or just tell them, "great work." They like to be complimented, too.

·   It's OK to get frustrated with them sometimes, or to want to play alone or with somebody else sometimes. We want to do that with our other friends, too.

·   Don't be afraid to ask them to do something. They are neat kids and can do a lot of things.

·   Find something to like, a special skill to admire, or a special interest they have. Some kids with Asperger Sydrome are great with Mad Minute in math, or they are great at spelling, or computers, or they have a great memory for the class schedule. If you can find that special thing, then you have something to admire about them.

While children are often willing to befriend a child with Asperger Syndrome, they need a certain amount of structure and encouragement to do so. Parents and professionals need to set the stage by providing good examples of how to treat people with disabilities, and by supporting the kids in their positive efforts.

As you help your child with Asperger Syndrome forge crucial connections, always keep in mind the lessons of these children, and of teammates on William's basketball team: When you help your child be part of things, when you help her build her skills, you are not just doing your child a service, but you're helping her bring her considerable gifts to others as well.

9

Generation "Why"

Adolescence: So Much to Learn, So Little Time

Tim's most fervent wish by the middle of freshman year was also his greatest challenge: He wanted a girlfriend. In our discussions, the concept of relationships was a black-and-white affair: You either had a girlfriend or you didn't. The notion of having a variety of friends, some girls and some boys, eluded him. What's more, the concept of showing interest in someone else in a friendly manner, but without romantic implications, was entirely foreign.

Starting high school had not been easy for Tim. His tendency to discuss police scanners, dispatching, and related topics was not valued by the other students, and his style of dress tended toward loose sweatpants and police or fire department T-shirts. He had trouble adjusting to the size of the high school and often became lost. Class bells hurt his ears, and his tendency to panic was only increased by the physical confusion in the hallways between classes. Tim sometimes perceived jostling or accidental bumping by classmates while at his locker as physical attacks.

The question of a girlfriend was revisited in his sophomore year. Two senior girls had learned of Tim's difficulty in school and were interested in helping him negotiate the social culture. They had lockers near his, and had frequent, casual contact with him before and after school. One day during one of our visits Tim informed me that one of the girls, Laura, was interested in him, and he was sure that she wanted to be his girlfriend (a prospect which pleased him greatly). The evidence he cited for this was her friendliness toward him, the fact that she liked police dispatching and scanners (evidenced by her listening to him talk about these), and that she always said hello to him in the hallways. What's more, when he had asked her if he could call her at home if he had a question about something in school, she said yes and gave him her phone number.

This motivated Tim in positive ways: He paid closer attention to grooming (especially combing his hair, using deodorant, and cleaning his glasses). He accompanied his cousin to the mall on a clothes-buying trip and returned with a more stylish wardrobe. He made more conscious attempts to ask follow-up questions of others in conversation, rather than turning the topic to his own interest so quickly.

But Tim was not able to understand Laura's friendliness as anything except romantic interest. Although she had a steady boyfriend, this didn't faze him. The fact that she went on dates weekly with her boyfriend, and was attending the Senior Prom with him, mattered little to Tim. He was certain that she would ultimately choose him over the other young man, because she was always so friendly and kind to him.

Tim began telephoning her more frequently. When she told him that her parents didn't want her to spend so much time on the phone, he started to e-mail her. Unanswered e-mails were re-sent the next day. Tim began to propose places to meet, or go out to dinner, through e-mail messages, but all were declined for one reason or another. Despite Tim's persistence, which became excessive, this thoughtful teenager remained pleasant and friendly toward Tim in school.

Eventually, she had to explain to Tim that their friendship was important to her, but that she didn't want it to be a "boyfriend-girl-friend" relationship. She reiterated that she had a boyfriend, and would be going off to college in September. Her gentle insistence allowed Tim to begin to understand the different nature of their relationship, and ultimately he was able to maintain their friendship on those terms for the remainder of the school year.

In discussing the issues with me, Tim observed that his first problem was that he had chosen someone who would be graduating before him. "That's the problem," he said. "If she had more time to get to know me, things might turn out differently."

Tim's difficulty with relationships illustrates what a struggle it can be for children with Asperger Syndrome to negotiate the perilous world of adolescence. The teen years are turbulent enough for typical children. But for kids like Tim, hazards—some obvious, some hidden—lurk around every corner. Romantic relationships, in particular, can be difficult for young people with Asperger Syndrome to negotiate, although their chances for fulfillment increase in adulthood.

Yet Tim has made progress. He entered high school looking and acting like an awkward little kid. He will graduate looking like a man, with many more social graces. Thanks to consistent support and the help of a kind young woman, Tim has learned something about relationships, has improved his grooming and his conversational skills, and has some experience communicating with the opposite sex.

In this chapter, we'll examine the particular challenges that your child will confront in adolescence, and outline guidelines for helping him emerge from adolescence as a more independent, more confident adult.

First, Recognize There's a Teen in There

Sometimes time gets away from us as parents. The years pass, and then something happens that jolts us into the realization that our child has moved on to a new stage of development. It may be the discovery of a sexually explicit magazine that startles us into the realization that our child is maturing. It may be an unprecedented resistance to going on a family vacation that he previously enjoyed.

Sometimes, it's the new abilities that surprise us. A child who has hesitated to go into a store on his own now asks for money and says he'll buy his own school supplies, or insists he can travel by himself to another city.

That happens in all families, of course, but parents of children with Asperger Syndrome can be lulled during preteen years because their children provide fewer warnings that adolescence is fast approaching.

Typical eleven- or twelve-year-olds often are eager to appear like teens or tiny adults; they may mimic adult and teen behavior before they've arrived chronologically.

A child with Asperger Syndrome, however, often is content to remain a child, to wear the same kinds of clothing, to play the same games, or tinker with the same hobbies.

But the same forces are at work, and suddenly your child stands before you, taller, stronger, with the shape of a woman or the beard of a young man. Suddenly, your child is arguing with you about everything, and arguing more effectively at that. He's more stubborn, less flexible than ever. He's quite certain that he knows more than his parents (and he may be right). He has an unrealistic sense of his own capabilities.

Like his peers, your child will feel pulled between his desire for independence on one hand, and his need for your guidance and support on the other. But your teenager with Asperger Syndrome is less able to be independent, at least at this stage. He still needs considerable help, even if he doesn't always accept it gracefully.

Like all teenagers, he will experience uncertainty about his identity, his future, his acceptability to others. He may be acutely aware of his social inadequacies. He's aware that he isn't getting all he wants out of life. He'd like a romantic connection, but has no idea how to go about it. He wants to drive, but may not be capable of doing so safely.

He may, like Tim, believe that if only he works harder, tries harder, he will overcome his troubles and overcome the resistance of others.

Basic Strategies for the Teen Years

Many of the same strategies that you've applied throughout your child's early years are still valid during adolescence, but with slightly different emphasis. Here are some examples.

Be clear and explicit about your expectations. Your child needs to know what you expect of him at home, at school, and in the community. Your rules—the ones he clung to as a child—may now be challenged. You will need to update and reinterpret rules so they are appropriate for his development, but you will still need rules—and he will still crave them. Clearly, curfews and limitations on where he goes will need to be discussed and adjusted as he demonstrates greater ability to take care of himself on his own.

You will need to continue to be explicit. If you want to stress the importance of grooming, you should not say, "You *do* want to get invited to the spring dance, don't you?" Instead, focus on the specific action: "It is important to take a shower every day and use deodorant. This makes people enjoy being around you."

Maintain predictability. Your child's need for sameness hasn't changed. Keep to family routines and schedules, and prepare your child for alterations in plans. What has changed is his readiness to use that foundation of security to develop a greater tolerance for change.

Expand flexibility. Your "What-if?" games of earlier years can become brainstorming sessions in which you talk about the situations your child might find himself in, and what behavior he should practice so he'll be able to manage. Continue to focus on safety and independence issues. Ask what your child would do if he got lost, was offered a ride in a stranger's car, and so on. Also, work on ways to expand and enlarge the routines that have offered comfort and stability to your child.

Expand responsibilities. Household chores, which may have been quite limited when your child was young, need to be expanded. Responsibility is beneficial for self-confidence and self-esteem. In addition, your child needs to continue to work on the life skills that will help him in adulthood. For example, he can take care of his clothes, tidy up the kitchen, or do other chores, but as before, he may need prompts and reminders. Lists and charts continue to be useful, as do photos of what a completed job should look like.

If possible, your child should be taking on some kind of responsibility outside the home, either paid employment or volunteer work. This experience not only builds confidence and self-esteem, but also provides essential experience of the world of work, in a real-world context. No amount of career training or classroom education will prepare a young person for work life the way an actual employment or volunteer experience does.

Essential Skills to Work On in the Teen Years

Leisure skills. It's important to develop activities and interests that provide enjoyment and opportunities to socialize. For some children, this might be a sport, a musical instrument, or an art class. Base activities on interests, and use interests to provide a setting for social skill-building. One young man who loves airplanes has joined a group of adult men who go out to the park every Saturday to fly remote control airplanes. He enjoys building and flying the planes, and the men accept him as a junior member of the group.

Conversation. Continue working on issues of turn-taking (to avoid monopolizing a conversation), asking for information, avoiding interruptions, and acknowledging interest in the other person's comments.

Interpreting the affective responses of others. Discuss facial expressions, indications of interest or boredom, signs of offense, and so on, and practice in areas in which your child needs extra help.

Humor. Discuss with your child ways to tell when someone is joking. Give him scripts for checking whether another person's comments were meant in jest or not ("You *are* joking, right?"). Enjoy his unique brand of humor and talk about what you and he find amusing. Many teenagers with Asperger Syndrome enjoy memorizing and reciting dialog from movies and television programs they find amusing (Monty Python movies are a favorite of several of my patients).

Accepting correction. Give criticism directly but tactfully. It's best to express it in terms of feedback, rather than criticism, because that emphasizes its positive, constructive aspect. Expect your child to get better at accepting suggestions and feedback without excess argument. This is a skill that everyone will need in adult life. The same thing applies to criticizing others as well. Provide a script for your child to use when he thinks someone is in error. This might include phrases like, "That might work, but I think this would work better," or "How about if we try this?"

Negotiation and compromise. Often children with Asperger Syndrome see the world in black and white. Help your child see that many situations are "gray areas" that other well-meaning people may interpret differently. For example, the difference between a regular lie and a "white lie" may be lost on him. Explain that the first is usually wrong, while the second is intended as a way to be kind.

Interpreting greetings and the appropriate responses. This would include making the distinction between "How are you," which calls for a simple, "Fine. How are you?" and something like "So, how was your trip to Hawaii?" which calls for more detail.

Interpreting put-downs. So much discourse among teenagers is slang, faddish, or sarcastic. Your child may choose to avoid such conversations, but it's helpful to teach him what they mean. For example, some kids say "You're so *bad!*" as a compliment.

Responding to authority figures. Practice with your child appropriate responses to school officials, police officers, security personnel at the mall, and others who may expect quick compliance.

Understanding and expressing one's own feelings. Encourage your child to talk about his feelings, when he can. Model phrases that address emotions—your own and his. "I've been acting kind of angry today because the garage can't seem to get my car fixed right," or "I think you're feeling a bit anxious about the test tomorrow." Encourage him to keep a journal and write down what's happening in his own emotional life.

Help Your Child Fit In Socially

"Academics were my life in high school," recalls a young woman with Asperger Syndrome. "That's how I survived day to day. I studied all the time. I felt the other kids didn't like me, and I didn't much want to hang around with them. All they wanted to talk about was boys and hair and shopping, and I wanted to talk about space and computers."

Looking back, this young woman (who wasn't diagnosed until early adulthood) thinks parents should try to help their children find a balance between pursuing their genuine interests, and building their social skills. Many teenagers with Asperger Syndrome do spend quite a bit of time alone, with their books or hobbies, rather than in social groups. To some extent, this is reasonable. However, if your child hunkers down in his room and insists other kids are "stupid" and "boring," there needs to be a balance between what is comfortable, and what helps him grow and develop.

"The social piece is really important," she says. "Some kids might not like associating with people, but it's a skill like learning how to read. You don't let a dyslexic kid refuse to read just because he doesn't feel like it."

Ideally, your teen has developed considerable social skills and some connections with other kids, either through supportive community activities and clubs, or through an Asperger Syndrome support group. But social errors will still occur from time to time, and your task is to continue to help with social skills and social understanding, and to help your child find and maintain a niche and a cohort of peers.

However, he may be acutely aware of the difference between his social life and that of other teens. He may feel the pain of not belonging to a particular group of kids. He may strike up conversations with someone he deems "popular," then—if that person talks to him—conclude that he is fully accepted.

Remind your child that the "in-crowd" popularity issue is transient, and those status issues often evaporate after high school. Remind him that you make friends by sharing an activity or interest; you don't just label somebody a friend (or girlfriend). Point out that he spends time with a great group of kids with whom he plays computer games, or has chess tournaments, or gets together for pizza to talk over Asperger issues. At the same time, keep working on helping your child fit in as much as possible. Help him find his niche, or develop it in more age-appropriate ways. An early interest in Legos may translate in adolescence into participating on a Lego Mindstorm Robotics Team. An interest in animals may lead to volunteer work at the local SPCA, or the animal rescue clinic at the local nature center. You can continue to seek mentors to support your child's interests, especially adolescents, older kids, and community members.

Computers can open a world of communication for children with Asperger Syndrome. E-mail and chat rooms provide an opportunity for articulate but awkward teens to communicate with others in a fairly low-stress way. Instant messaging is a popular way for typical teens to communicate, and kids with Asperger Syndrome can join in those conversations with considerable ease.

It's important to teach your child the basic safety rules about using the Internet. As with all your rules, be specific and clear-cut. Tell your child not to give out personal information, such as his full name, in chat rooms, and not to share identifying information about himself or his family with anyone he meets on-line.

Some protection can be provided by blocking software, like Cyber Patrol, but ultimately parental supervision and monitoring are essential for your child's safety.

A Matter of Style

Now is the time to encourage your child to look his age. Clothes and grooming are often big issues for all adolescents, but typical teens usually err in favor of slavishly following fads and fashions. For kids with Asperger Syndrome, the problem is usually just the opposite. They don't notice changing conventions as quickly as others, or may prefer a style of clothing because it is very familiar or more comfortable due to sensory challenges. Like Tim, they may wear the same style of baggy sweatpants they've worn since first grade. Try to help your child stay current. To do this, you may want to enlist a shopping buddy—perhaps a friend or cousin—to help choose appropriate clothing.

Hygiene and grooming are major issues. Many kids with Asperger Syndrome resist showering, shaving, or using deodorant. They may resist because of the sensory issues we've discussed earlier. They may argue that they don't see the need, or choose not to bother with such trivialities. They may be so disorganized in the morning that they don't get it together sufficiently for these tasks to be accomplished.

These grooming basics, however, will need to be non-negotiable if your child is to be accepted socially. Develop a "grooming and personal hygiene" checklist for the mornings. The checklist can include a picture of how "the total package" should look (shoes tied, shirt in or out, zippers zipped, and so on). If you have difficulty getting through in your role as parent, again try to enlist a buddy or mentor to help.

When your child looks presentable, praise his appearance. As he takes more responsibility for these adult tasks, praise his progress toward maturity.

All's Fair

As we saw with Alison, whom we met at the beginning of chapter 7 as she argued about the algebra quiz, the volatile combination of Asperger Syndrome and adolescence can bring out extremes of rigidity about rules, about what's fair, and how things *should* be done.

Often, adolescents with Asperger Syndrome become more rigid, just at a point in their lives when they would benefit from a bit more flexibility. Yet this stage is developmentally sound: typical adolescents often become much more interested in issues of right and wrong, on a broader scale than when they were children. They become more idealistic and interested in ethical issues. So it's not surprising that your teen might become a "rule enforcer," both at home and at school.

Teenagers with Asperger Syndrome have difficulty with the idea that you can be right and wrong at the same time. You may be right about a particular rule, but absolutely wrong about its relative importance, or the appropriateness of the time and place that you bring it up, or about the impact it has on others. Kids with Asperger Syndrome often expect that their legalistic attachment to rules will bring them praise, when in reality the opposite is true. As Temple Grandin put it, for people with Asperger Syndrome, "Rules are very important, because we concentrate intensely on how things are done." One thing she had to learn was that "being technically right is not always socially right."

When you discuss the rules/fairness issue with your child, make the point that fairness does not mean that everybody gets the same thing. It means that everybody should get what they need.

For example, your child might get extra time to complete a test, or be allowed to dictate the answer to an essay question, or use a word processor to write because cursive is so laborious. Other students don't get these adaptations and accommodations. That's OK, because your child needs them, while others do not.

You can use this kind of example to point out that fair and unfair are not always obvious, and depend on context and circumstances. And reiterate that just because someone doesn't always follow the rules does not mean that they are bad, or unworthy of respect.

You can also remind your child about "rules" of etiquette and diplomacy. Even though someone may be violating a particular rule, it may be kinder or more appropriate to let it go without comment. After all, tact and consideration for the feelings of others are among the rules of etiquette. Encourage your teenager to hold off on pouncing on other people's failings. He might wait, ask you, sleep on it, and then decide whether the issue is worth a confrontation.

Relationships and Sexuality

As the parent of a child with Asperger Syndrome, you have undoubtedly worried about how your child will negotiate the complex realm of sexuality. It's not just the matter of popularity, or making friends, that is of concern. There's the whole matter of your child's safety, as well as his ability to avoid offending others. Your salvation, in this realm, is that your child is capable, and enthusiastic, about rules. Therefore, you will need to teach issues of sexuality, safety, and relationships very explicitly.

Relationships. It's important for all teens to understand that not every teenager has a girlfriend or boyfriend. Many go contentedly through their high school years with friends of the same gender, or by spending time with groups of both boys and girls rather than having an actual romantic partner.

Teenagers with Asperger Syndrome are less likely than other teens to date and have romantic relationships during their high school years. Many are content to spend time alone or with one friend, or to take part in group activities. Some, like Tim, would very much like to have a girlfriend but do not have the social understanding and maturity to make that happen. Also, not all boyfriend/girlfriend relationships involve sexual activity. A satisfying relationship may include companionship, affection, and pleasure in the company of an appealing person, but nothing more.

It is important to stress that in order to learn how to be a boyfriend or girlfriend, you must first learn how to be a friend. It's important to be explicit about what friendship involves, because teenagers with Asperger Syndrome may have few friends, and limited group experience, from which to draw these lessons. Point out that many of the same social skills, such as conversation and spending time at shared leisure activities, apply to same-sex and opposite-sex relationships. These may, in the future, lead to a different or more committed relationship, or they may not, but either way, the child with Asperger Syndrome will have expanded social opportunities and have newly developed skills in place when opportunities present themselves.

Not all children with Asperger Syndrome are eager for social interaction, but many are. In one support group for teenagers, the kids (who attended several different high schools) decided to invite one another to their proms. In this way, they were able to participate, and also to be assured that the evening would be relatively comfortable because they attended with another person whom they already knew, and who shared some of their interests.

The line between showing interest and harassment. It is critical to make sure your child understands this distinction, and the distinction between friendly interest and excess interest. As we saw in Tim's situation, young people with Asperger Syndrome can be very determined in their pursuit of a relationship. While the ability to stick to a goal without giving up is admirable, it can sometimes lead to difficulties. Be very explicit in explaining to your child the difference between "being friendly," "showing interest," and outright stalking. Explain why people can become upset and even frightened when the pursuit is too intense or prolonged. Try to help your child understand that every show of friendship from another person does not necessarily mean that the person is romantically interested.

It may be helpful to use the definition for sexual harassment as a benchmark for inappropriate behavior. If your child's school has a sexual harassment policy for students (and most do) review it with your child and make it a point of discussion both in your home and in your child's support or therapy groups. Point out the behaviors—unwanted staring, inappropriate comments, following, touching—that are unacceptable, and why.

Be sure to test your child to be sure he understands the rules in context. One college student learned in freshman orientation the lessons about date rape and harassment a bit too well: Rule was, if a man wishes to touch a woman's body, he must ask for permission. The young man proceeded to walk up to young women on campus and ask if he could touch them.

Others have run into trouble because of their literal interpretation of language. If a young man is admiring a woman's body, and she glares at him and says, "What are *you* looking at?" he may well offend her when he tells her plainly what he is looking at. Both boys and girls need to know and expand on the rules about "good touch, bad touch." They need to know that "no means no" when someone else says it, and that their own "no means no" as well.

Here again, your child's fondness for following rules will help him apply these guidelines. When he does misbehave, remember that kids with Asperger Syndrome usually do so because they don't know what to do, or misunderstood the rules. It's far more effective to deal with lapses using Social Autopsies (chapter 8) and a discussion of acceptable alternatives, than punishing or shaming. Despite the miserable title, the book *Dating for Dummies* can be a good reference guide.

Sexuality. This can be a minefield for kids (and adults) with Asperger Syndrome, in part, because of the innuendo, euphemism, and double meanings rampant in the way we talk about sexuality. It's crucial that your child be taught explicitly about sex, and about how his body functions. Winks and nudges, or allegories about birds and bees, will not work. Most middle schools have units on sexuality and health. Keep close contact with your school on this issue, and be sure to reinforce at home lessons about sexually transmitted diseases, contraception, and the use of condoms.

Computer-literate kids with Asperger Syndrome (and that's most of them) have no doubt discovered erotic or pornographic sites. Pornography is entirely inappropriate as a teaching guide, because all too often it contains inappropriate themes—power and submission, degradation, and sometimes violence. As we suggested earlier, make use of parental controls and Web site–locking technology, but reinforce that with ongoing discussions about healthy sexuality.

You will need to explain to your child that the sex lives of most people are not like sexual activity as portrayed in pornography. As a source of sexuality education pornography is, thus, not appropriate. If explicit information seems advised for older students, serious "marital aids" videos are vastly preferable.

The issue of privacy about sexual matters must be stressed. Emphasize that privacy applies both to your child and to other people. Masturbation—both in terms of the "when and where" issues and strategies—should be taught explicitly. If the same-sex parent isn't available, a relative or friend needs to be recruited for this important task.

As a cautionary tale, let me offer the story of a patient of mine. As a young man, Bob became very interested in weight lifting. His mother was dead, and his father was ill, so he had less guidance than he needed during these crucial years. Through a family member he met a terrific man, an attorney, who took a personal (and completely appropriate) interest in helping him.

Knowing of Bob's interest in fitness, the attorney took him to his own gym, and this event became a weekly activity for them both. Bob eventually joined the gym on his own. Once, after a workout, the attorney went for a massage at the gym, and Bob said he'd like to try it. He did, and he liked it.

Later, the masseuse left the gym and wasn't replaced. Months went by, and one day Bob noticed an ad in an alternative weekly newspaper for massages (in the adult section of the paper). Bob decided to go for a massage there. He was greeted in the lobby by a woman who asked for his credit card for payment. Bob complied, and was led into a small room with a bed, occupied by a nude woman, who attempted to undress him.

Bob was not expecting this at all, and ran from the establishment in a panic, forgetting his credit card. He got home and called his attorney friend, who told him to go back for the card. Unfortunately, someone had already run up several thousand dollars worth of charges on the card. The situation was ultimately resolved without Bob paying any money, but the risk he placed himself in inadvertently was substantial—not to mention the emotional upset and embarrassment he experienced.

Had Bob been a teenager, his naive behavior might have been more understandable. But as a man in his late twenties, his innocence went beyond what is typical. While the situation Bob faced may appear unlikely to a parent at first, consider the trust your child sometimes places in others who appear in authority, and where that naiveté may lead if he isn't taught or guided.

Anxiety and Emotions

One of my patients, Ryan, suffered from anxiety in ways that are typical of adolescents with Asperger Syndrome. He tended to worry obsessively about a range of events, from difficulties at school to burglars or fires at home. At seventeen, he dreaded being home by himself, so he spent many hours at his parents' office, across the street from the municipal building.

Although Ryan was highly sensitive to noises, he handled them well when they were predictable. The loud bell that tolled the hours on the municipal clock tower across from his parents' office became a soothing ritual for Ryan—until the day the clock broke down.

The bell rang erratically, and sometimes skipped an hour entirely. It took weeks before maintenance workers could get it fixed, and during this time, Ryan became increasingly agitated to the point that his school work suffered and his social skills regressed.

A variety of cognitive-behavioral strategies proved helpful with Ryan. We gave a specific limit on the number of telephone calls he could make to the city about when the clock would be fixed. We had him use other timepieces (not the municipal clock) to check the time. And we gave him specific relaxation and distraction techniques to ease his anxiety.

Like Ryan, your adolescent may worry excessively or be subject to panic attacks. Other emotional difficulties of adolescents with Asperger Syndrome are less obvious.

Depression, in particular, is a risk among teenagers with Asperger Syndrome. Any child who feels helpless, hopeless, and isolated can become depressed. According to the National Institute of Mental Health, as many as 8 percent of all adolescents in the United States suffer from depression. Although statistics are not available, professionals believe that the incidence is much higher among young people with Asperger Syndrome.

Adolescent depression in general is often not recognized because symptoms of unhappiness are often attributed to the normal miseries of adolescence. In children with Asperger Syndrome, recognition is more difficult because these children often do not express their unhappiness in typical ways. For this reason, it's essential to stay attuned to your child's emotional well-being. It's helpful if your son or daughter has been seeing a counselor regularly.

Symptoms of major depressive disorder in typical populations of adults and adolescents are:

- persistent sad or irritable mood
- loss of interest in activities once enjoyed
- significant change in appetite or body weight
- difficulty sleeping, or oversleeping

· psychomotor agitation or retardation
· loss of energy
· feelings of worthlessness or inappropriate guilt
· difficulty concentrating
· recurrent thoughts of death or suicide

Five or more of these symptoms must be present for at least two weeks before a diagnosis of major depression is indicated.

Signs associated with depression in adolescents are:

· frequent or vague, nonspecific physical complaints such as headaches, muscle aches, stomachaches, or tiredness
· frequent absences from school or poor performance in school
· talk of or efforts to run away from home
· outbursts of shouting, complaining, unexplained irritability, or crying
· being bored
· lack of interest in playing with friends
· alcohol or substance abuse
· social isolation, poor communication
· fear of death
· extreme sensitivity to rejection or failure
· increased irritability, anger, or hostility
· reckless behavior
· difficulty with relationships

The recovery rate from a single episode of depression is high. Antidepressant medications, especially when combined with cognitive behavior therapy and family therapy, can be very effective treatments for depression. For individuals with Asperger Syndrome, the more concrete "here-and-now" problem-solving emphasis of cognitive behavior therapy can be quite useful.

For people with Asperger Syndrome, the clinical signs of depression may be similar to those listed, but they may be different. What's important to recognize are sudden (and significant) changes in behavior, and whether those changes persist. Self-imposed isolation, negative and destructive thoughts and verbalizations, and any talk of suicide or of the hopelessness of life must be brought to the attention of a qualified mental health professional immediately, preferably one who has experience with individuals with Asperger Syndrome.

Driving

The driver's license is a key to adulthood for typical teenagers. For some teens with Asperger Syndrome the issue is not a problem: they are able to cope well, with adequate training.

For many, however, a whole series of difficulties arises. Stressful traffic situations can send anxiety and stress sky high. The lack of predictability adds a level of difficulty. And the whole issue of judgment and executive function comes into play. Defensive driving calls for the ability to put oneself in another driver's position, and to imagine what someone else might do—and to do all of this instantaneously.

Thus, although driving is important as an independence issue, it must be viewed foremost as a safety issue. Just as your child learned to cross the street safely (but perhaps later than other children), he may be able to learn to drive safely, but perhaps later than other teens. If you take this approach, be sure that your child has access to plenty of driver training and driver education. Your state's rehabilitation agency may be able to provide a list of driving instructors that specialize in adaptive lessons for people who have a range of disabilities, including anxiety.

If you are fortunate enough to live near adequate public transportation, teach your child to cope with the complexities of schedules, exact change, tokens, transfers, and the inevitable delays. As we've seen, an interest in trains and buses is not unusual; your child may well enjoy learning the mechanics of travel on public transport.

It's the less tangible skills he'll have to practice, however. He'll need to know what to do when the bus is late, or when there's another emergency. He'll even need to learn unspoken etiquette of transportation: if the train or bus is not crowded, you generally leave space between yourself and other passengers, rather than sit down right next to them. You don't generally strike up a conversation. If the bus doesn't come, you can either wait for the next one or call home, and so on.

Education

Higher education is a realistic goal for many young people with Asperger Syndrome. But the experiences of people who do go on to college and graduate school vary. For some, the larger setting of a college, and the degree of independence expected of college students, may be too much unless they are able to obtain support.

As you and your child consider college options, carefully review what support each school will offer your child. Contact the college's Division of Disability Support, or equivalent office established to ensure appropriate adaptations and accommodations to people with disabilities. Federal law guarantees that otherwise qualified students must be given the extra assistance required by their disability if needed to pursue their studies.

These accommodations may include, among other things, extra time for test-taking, note-taking assistance, and single room accommodations. Many schools have dormitories with specific requirements, such as "quiet" dorms, no smoking/drinking dorms, and so on. These placements often suit someone with sensory issues, or who is upset and offended by the rowdy behavior that's so much a part of dormitory life.

The school may assign a counselor to help your child negotiate the maze of college, and perhaps help with organization of work, much as a resource room teacher helped in public school. Many schools have a "big sister/little sister" (or brother) program for all new students, in which an older student takes a younger one under wing and remains available as a mentor or helper throughout the year.

Some young adults with Asperger Syndrome report that their transition from home to college was eased by selecting a small, nurturing school, or by attending a same-sex institution. Both these settings reduce the social demands placed on a young student.

Getting extra help in college is not unusual, by the way, and not limited to people with disabilities. For example, consider the academic support counselors that many universities employ for members of athletic teams who might otherwise have difficulty maintaining their academic schedules during the school year. The important thing is to be clear about assistance needed when selecting a college or university, and to discuss these issues in advance with admission officers.

Dania Jekel, a social worker who serves as executive director of the Asperger's Association of New England, has worked with numerous adolescent and adult support groups. She suggests the following guidelines for young people with Asperger Syndrome planning for college:

1. Be open about the diagnosis, and what support you will need from the college.
2. Select a college at least in part on the basis of how supportive it will be.
3. Consider a college that is near home, or consider living at home the first year.
4. Consider a single room, or a single room that's part of a suite.
5. Don't take too heavy a course schedule. You might take a reduced course load the first year.
6. Use whatever support is available, particularly when it comes to organizing assignments, and organizing your time.

"Things Get Better After High School"

Try to stay upbeat as you and your adolescent with Asperger Syndrome struggle through the teen years. One way to do that is to remind your child, and yourself, that things often improve in the lives of people with Asperger Syndrome when they move beyond the peer-group pressure cooker of the junior high and high school years. As children grow older, so do their peers, and by early adulthood, much less teasing goes on.

In later life, as we'll see in the next chapter, your young adult will have more choices about how to spend time, less pressure to do things he finds objectionable, and more chances to spend his time as he chooses. In short, there's less algebra and more penguins.

Because of earlier efforts by you and his teachers, your child will also have greater social skills, and be more able to downplay those aspects of his Asperger Syndrome that drew unfavorable attention when he was younger. He will receive more honor and respect for those subjects where he is knowledgeable; while not every teenager is interested in police scanners, there are volunteer rescue squads where everyone will be impressed with Tim's knowledge.

And the nature of friendship and relationships changes as people mature. Trying to keep up with ever-changing fashion and break into social groups is tough for Asperger Syndrome teenagers. Once they reach adulthood, that aspect of life and "popularity" recedes a bit. As your child gets older, he will find more people who appreciate the kinds of qualities so typical in young adults with Asperger Syndrome: intelligence, rational thinking, honesty, and integrity.

10

The World Beyond

Your Child as an Adult

All parents dream about their children's future life, and for all parents, those dreams sometimes include anxious moments. Will my child succeed? Be a good neighbor and citizen? Find friendship and love and family?

As the parent of a child with Asperger Syndrome, your dreams and worries are influenced by the reality that your child has a lifelong disability. By the time your child approaches adolescence, you have seen how the condition has presented challenges to your child in terms of relationships, academics, organization, planning—all the areas that we associate with adult independence.

As we have said, Asperger Syndrome doesn't go away. You don't cure it. And yet, this condition in adulthood presents a brighter picture than one might think. In this chapter, we'll look at what you can expect as your child embarks on a more independent life, what help she will still need, and what her future may hold. People with developmental disabilities, and those who work with them, refer to this stage as transition—a milestone, and an ongoing process, that marks the shift from dependency and childhood to independence and adulthood.

By the time your child reaches adolescence, you know a great deal about her, about Asperger Syndrome, and about the strengths and weaknesses it brings to your child's experience. By the time your child is an adult, both of you will know much more. Here are the thoughts of a mother, as she imagines her adolescent son's future:

> I believe that Jeremy can look forward to a bright future. Although he hasn't focused on what he might like to do for his life's work, patterns of interest are shaping up. The support of the computer as a communication tool will figure heavily into his choices.
>
> Even though they say kids with Asperger Syndrome don't show much empathy, the care and concern that Jeremy showed me during a recent illness certainly feels like love and empathy to me . . . He knows how to show and receive love and understands when he has done something to hurt someone's feelings. He says he's sorry and makes amends. He's beginning to choose friends who have the strengths that he doesn't have.
>
> I am sure that he will find a life partner. He's an interesting character who will attract other interesting people.

You are well qualified to launch your child into the adult world, just as all parents hope to launch their children. Most of what you and your child need to do at this point is a natural extension of what you have done throughout your child's life, and what we have discussed throughout this book. And the goal that you both should keep in mind at all times is independence. Whether your child is completely independent and self-supporting, or needs some assists along the way, the more independent she can be, the more fulfilling her life will be.

For example, your adult child will need to take on the role of advocacy for herself. When she needs help, she will need to ask for it more and more on her own. But that advocacy role is one that you began years ago, when you first explained your child's behavior or diagnosis to others. From the beginning, you fed and dressed your child and took responsibility for her health and well-being. Later, you arranged her social life and advocated for her educational rights. Over time, you have transferred elements of this responsibility to your child, and in so doing fostered her independence.

The same lifelong process—and transfer of power—occurs in other areas. We never stop being parents, whether our child has a disability or not. As parents, we want our adult children to be happy and fulfilled, but we know they will need to achieve happiness and fulfillment without us some day. We also hope that our children will find other sources of support in their lives. If we have other children, we hope that they and other family members will to some extent look after our less able child, as will the extended family. But in the immediate future, you will stay involved in the life of your child with Asperger Syndrome. Your role will become less hands-on and more advisory, but it will continue.

Parents and family have an enormous impact on how well people with Asperger Syndrome develop, and thus how able they are to lead successful lives as adults. Parents need to be reminded of this important fact, especially because people with Asperger Syndrome may not be good at expressing their feelings.

The daunting task of launching your child can seem more manageable if it's viewed as a process, another stage in the foundation you and your child have been building for years.

The Essential Elements of Transition

For all children, adolescence marks a major—and often difficult—passage from childhood to adulthood. A young adult of eighteen is hardly a polished specimen of maturity. Maturation will continue throughout life, although most young people sort out the key issues of adulthood while they are in their twenties. These include determining career choices and making preparations for a career; determining the kind of relationships one seeks, both in love and friendship; and determining what kind of values one will pursue and support.

Employment

Clearly, a decent job is the key to adult independence. The ability to find a market for one's talents and skills, to receive a regular paycheck, and to pay one's way in society is essential to our concept of adult independence.

The good news is that many people with Asperger Syndrome have two key advantages as they search for work. First, they often have considerable strengths in certain areas. Usually, it's the "unusual interest" that evolves into a field of study or expertise. Tim, with his interest in police scanners, might enter a technical aspect of law enforcement, or learn to design or repair electronic equipment. Alison, with her interest in waterfowl, may pursue a career in biology or ornithology (and perhaps write her dissertation on the molting habits of various penguins).

Trains, meteorology, medieval society, aviation—throughout this book we have noted the rather amazing subjects that may capture the attention of children with Asperger Syndrome. It's not essential that your child's career choices revolve around an intense interest, but often such an interest will point the way.

Of course, the passion itself doesn't necessarily lead to realistic career plans. One young woman who was passionate about space and astronomy was hoping to become an astronaut, but later realized that perhaps being blasted off into space might not be a good career move for someone who struggles with anxieties and sensory issues.

Beyond the specific interest itself, many people with Asperger Syndrome have strengths in mathematics, in memory, and in linear, logical thinking—all of which are at a premium in the workplace. The bad news is that adults with Asperger Syndrome often are underemployed, or working in areas that don't capitalize on those strengths. The reasons are varied. They include sensitivity to noisy or fast-paced workplaces, difficulties with social relationships, and problems with social communication. An unspoken job qualification for so many kinds of employment is the ability to communicate—to give and receive instructions, stay in touch with coworkers and people from other departments, and converse easily with clients or customers.

And there are the more subtle aspects of workplace communication: the casual banter around the water cooler, the inside jokes, the subtle (and not-so-subtle) put-downs of bosses and coworkers. Good-natured banter is a big part of many offices, and has gotten many typical workers into hot water when jokes or innocently intended flirtations are misinterpreted. Imagine, then, the minefield that this presents for an employee with Asperger Syndrome. Some get into awkward situations; others withdraw into their cubicles and avoid social interaction.

Job interviews, in particular, are difficult and can provide a roadblock for an applicant who is otherwise qualified. Applicants may panic (or fear they will panic) under pressure. They agonize over what to disclose to their potential employer about their condition. One young woman prepared for weeks for a major interview, and felt confident that she would be able to make a good impression. She had asked for specifics about the interview process, and had been told that two executives would be present. When she walked into the room on the morning of the interview, she saw three people, rather than the two she expected. Her confidence evaporated; she was barely able to speak, and she didn't get the offer despite her qualifications.

Even if hired, the employee with Asperger Syndrome may have difficulty negotiating office politics, customer contact, and a fast-paced or disorganized work environment. Often, adults with Asperger Syndrome who attempt to negotiate the workplace without adequate mentoring or support wind up seriously underemployed, working at jobs significantly below their capacity.

Let's examine the checkered career of Ted, who has had both successes and failures in his employment history. At forty-four, Ted lives with his elderly mother. He graduated from a New York state university with a degree in mathematics, which has always been his area of strength. He has earned a master's degree in mathematics, and is completing a second master's degree in accounting. He has passed two of the national accounting exams so far.

He had trouble getting jobs earlier in his career, because his awkwardness and social peculiarities meant that his job interviews were rarely a success. He ultimately took a volunteer position in the billing department of a local hospital, where he did very well. He moved on to become a bank teller, where he had trouble relating to the clientele successfully. He then became a window teller for Off-Track Betting, which turned out to be a disaster because the job required dealing with people under pressure at a frantic pace just before race time.

Then he found a job reviewing contracts for a major rental car company. Here he found his niche. He worked in relative isolation, caught many errors, and saved the company a great deal of money. He was named employee of the month many times. But when the car rental company merged, he lost his job and was unemployed for several months. Since then, he has been unable to find a good job, but is working—considerably below his abilities—as a motel night auditor/desk manager.

It's clear from Ted's employment history that he was successful in settings where he could do his work on his own, free of distractions and the stress of dealing with a parade of unfamiliar people. For people with Asperger Syndrome, there needs to be a good fit between the job and the person's abilities. What Ted needs is a mentor, or career counselor specializing in people with disabilities, who can help him network and identify employment opportunities and sympathetic employers. He needs ways of approaching potential employers and persuading them that accommodating his needs will enable him to be a highly productive member of the team.

There are such supports available. Most states have a Department of Rehabilitative Services, or equivalent, that offers some job training or coaching for people with disabilities. In addition, books on career selection (with self-assessment tests) can help a young adult with Asperger Syndrome narrow down suitable careers (see the Resources section).

A crucial element is the flexibility of the employer. As we see from Ted's experience, people with Asperger Syndrome can make excellent employees, and ought to be in demand on their merits alone. Sometimes, all it takes is an understanding and thoughtful mentor to help blaze—and maintain—the trail.

People with Asperger Syndrome tend to do best in technical, scholarly, or creative fields. In most cases, they thrive in pursuits that allow them to work independently and be recognized for their abilities, rather than for their social skills. Jobs that require a great deal of face-to-face interaction with the public, especially under stress, would be difficult. Many retail jobs, and positions in sales, are particularly difficult. Working as an airline ticketing agent might be the ultimate bad fit for most employees with Asperger Syndrome.

Management and sales jobs are often the most difficult. One young man who was a computer whiz had great difficulty in a job selling computers. He knew all about the technology, but couldn't handle the company's pressure to make the sale, whether the system was right for the customer or not. "They ask me to lie," he says. "They'll be pushing a particular computer, and I know it's not the right one for this person." And he can't lie, so he hasn't been successful.

People with Asperger Syndrome have found other careers to be promising, because they tend to be analytic and predictable, and minimize stressful social interactions:

- engineering
- biological research
- library science
- bookkeeping
- academic research (usually in nonteaching roles)
- music
- accounting
- veterinary science
- computer design
- information technology

In addition, some may find that self-employment matches their goals and their abilities. Often the reliability and integrity of the adult with Asperger Syndrome translates into success in a small business that does not require too much social interaction.

As we said in chapter 9, career planning and preparation should begin well before adulthood. Summer or part-time jobs during high school offer invaluable experience for all kids, but especially for young people with Asperger Syndrome. There's nothing like hands-on, specific experience to help develop job skills.

Mentoring

Your child with Asperger Syndrome will benefit from establishing relationships with adults who share a particular skill or interest. Often, these connections can be linked to your child's area of expertise or interest. Thus, the child who loves to read and established rapport with librarians may later volunteer to shelve books at the library, and establish a friendship with a member of the staff. A satisfying job may be the result of these efforts.

As your child enters adulthood, more than one mentor may be identified. There may be a job/career mentor, established around career interests or internships, and a community mentor, such as a clergy person or community agency worker, who can help identify and access community resources. Mentorship can develop in other areas, as well, but it all begins with a person who recognizes your child's uniqueness, and celebrates it as you do.

Mentoring can include such tasks as helping a supervisor or coworker work with the employee who has Asperger Syndrome. For example, a supervisor could be presented with a list of ways to communicate effectively with the employee. They might include, "Give assignments in writing," for example, or "Handle daily communication through e-mail." The supervisor could be advised to avoid phrases like "Get back to me on the double," and say instead, "Please give this to me by Thursday morning."

Continuing Education

Because so many people with Asperger Syndrome are capable of superior performance in academic work (with suitable accommodations), it is not uncommon for them to pursue advanced degrees. You and your child may have addressed the issue of college during her high school years. Whether she attended college or not, she, like many adults with Asperger Syndrome, may consider continuing her education, either for career training, starting a bachelor's program as an adult, or continuing with postgraduate study.

Some adults with Asperger Syndrome who find a niche in a university setting may pursue multiple degrees and still wind up underemployed. The ivory tower may be a comfortable setting, but is not ideal if the adult is never able to become independent and employed.

Living Arrangements

Where to live in adulthood is an intensely personal decision. Many adults with Asperger Syndrome continue to live with their families, receive support and companionship at home, and do well. For others, this is neither desirable nor possible. Ultimately, parents need to consider how and where their children will live when they are no longer able to provide support.

Thus, it's essential to consider other options, even if your child is likely to live at home. Other possibilities include living alone in an apartment or living with a roommate or roommates, with varying degrees of supervision. In some communities, partial supervision or "check-in" supports are available for adults with disabilities. This approach allows the adult to live independently with just enough supervision to make sure food shopping is done, bills are paid, and the person is generally managing. Disability organizations, local specialists in Asperger Syndrome, or self-advocacy and support groups can be instrumental in locating these resources.

Decisions about where to live are affected by the adult's ability to drive or use public transportation. The ability to drive is a crucial part of adult independence in most parts of the country. Ultimately, transportation skills—whether by car or alternate transit—will define the degree of independence your adult child will have.

Many adults with Asperger Syndrome are able to drive safely once they've had enough practice, but if driving is out of the question, the need for reliable public transportation will affect living arrangements and the decision about where to live. A city with an excellent rapid transit system is one likelihood, as are smaller towns with enlightened or imaginative paratransit or Ride-Share programs. If your child is unable to drive because of a disability, she is entitled to the use of subsidized transport systems.

Developing "Communities of Care"

Ideally, your child should be able to have some level of independence that goes beyond what the family is able or willing to provide. That's why, throughout this book, we've emphasized the importance of integrating your child into the outside community through athletics, organizations, and religious and community groups.

It is in these community organizations, whether religious or civic, and in local government agencies, that you will find the more formal support that will benefit your adult child. Even family friends can serve as mentors and resource persons and help your child be independent.

It's best when these supports are accomplished at the community level, because local grassroots support is more enduring than federal or state-mandated programs. They are less likely to be bureaucratic and legalistic, and more likely to be creative and innovative. Even in large urban communities, someone in a neighborhood association or apartment building association can identify or coordinate those services. You will do well to help your child identify these groups, and help her network with community leaders, to ensure some level of continuity in her community.

Self-Advocacy and Support

No one knows what it's like to have Asperger Syndrome, and what supports are helpful and available, as well as another person with Asperger Syndrome. Today there are numerous support groups, advocacy organizations, and Internet sources where young adults with Asperger Syndrome can turn for information and support.

Support groups also provide a much needed opportunity to socialize in a setting where one is understood—and one's limitations are understood. Help your child find them, and encourage participation if she finds the support helpful. Adults with Asperger Syndrome report that they feel a sense of empathy for other adults that is difficult for them to sense with others. They are among kindred spirits, people who understand. Group activity and discussion can do much more than provide support—it can be part of your child's continuing development of skills.

Not all adults will choose this route, and some may drop in and out of such groups as they feel inclined. "Initially, I found support groups helpful," one woman in her twenties told me. "I haven't been recently, though. Sometimes it isn't appealing to me that you're meeting on the basis of Asperger Syndrome. There are times when I'd rather meet with people because we're interested in the same things. But I wouldn't discourage someone from going."

Your Child as an Adult

The world today is a more welcoming place for people with Asperger Syndrome than it was a generation ago. A better understanding of Asperger Syndrome is only a few decades old, so today's adults with this condition spent their childhoods without the kinds of interventions that we now know are so helpful. So when we discuss the difficulties of adults, we can temper our concern with the knowledge that many of today's children are likely to do better, and become more capable adults. As time goes by, we will learn more about how adults with Asperger Syndrome cope at all stages of life, and we'll know more about what helps and what hinders them.

It is not going to be easy for your child to forge an independent life, but for many children, it will be a realizable goal. Your adult child will have legal supports that weren't there before, will have access to community services, and will take her place in a community that is more aware and accommodating of disabilities and diversity of all kinds.

British psychologist Digby Tantam, who has interviewed many adults with Asperger Syndrome, has found that the change from adolescence toward adulthood can be stressful and problematic because Asperger Syndrome produces deficits that are relatively mild and allow the adult to be "within reach" of a typical life yet not attain it. Young adults may suffer from seeing their peers enjoy many aspects of the transition to adulthood that they themselves find so difficult: enjoying more independence, getting jobs, furnishing their own apartments.

In addition, adulthood means that one's social and work focus becomes directed at peers. Often as children, people with Asperger Syndrome have been able to avoid direct head-on dealings with peers by interacting with other generations—either with adults or with much younger children, both of whom are more tolerant of their eccentricities. In adulthood, it becomes essential to interact with other adults in the workplace, in education, in housing, and in social settings.

However, it's important to keep in mind that many adults with Asperger Syndrome become vastly more able than they appeared in childhood and adolescence. Some traits, especially those relating to hypersensitivity, may ease in adulthood. Others, like anxiety, may ease with experience and maturity.

According to Tantam, it's quite common for adolescents and young adults to make rapid improvements in their social functioning. And these skills continue to mature and develop throughout adulthood. It's not clear yet precisely what causes this improvement, but a factor that appears to help considerably is peer interaction. One thing is true, however: The more your adult child is able to interact and be part of a community, the greater her skills are likely to become.

Finally, the world of adulthood offers everyone more choice in how they will live, and more control over the settings and situations in which they find themselves. They can decide what kind of work to do, where to live, who to associate with. Whatever eccentric interests and behaviors they may have, become, in the adult word, part of the vast range of human variation.

Love and Marriage

We've seen how challenging love, dating, and intimate relationships are for people with Asperger Syndrome. That challenge continues to some degree in adulthood. It's certainly a concern of parents, because we want our children to be happy and fulfilled. But what can we expect?

Here are the recollections of the parents of one child on learning that he had Asperger Syndrome: "When the diagnosis was rendered, we were numb at first. It was especially hard for his father to hear the psychiatrist explain that a child with Asperger Syndrome who grows up to be an adult with Asperger Syndrome will probably have a radically different take on what it means to be in love. Much of the intimacy and magic we associate with the constellation of emotions we call love may be absent or understood differently.

"Yes, we were told, someone will accept our son and love him as he is. Someone, perhaps, just like us?"

One young woman with Asperger Syndrome recalls how she met her husband at a New Year's Eve party. "I didn't go there planning to meet anybody," she said. "I was just planning to work on my social skills. I'd been trying to push myself socially." She met her husband, and found they shared interests in computers, books, and sailing. They married several years later.

In the typical world, love and marriage are expressed and arranged in a wide range of ways. Some people forge loving, stable relationships; others divorce and remarry several times. Some people remain single. People with Asperger Syndrome mirror this range, although they are somewhat less likely to marry.

However, adults with Asperger Syndrome who do find a stable relationship are often loyal and reliable partners. The very deficits that make relationship difficult—difficulty with empathy and understanding the subtle feelings of another—are counteracted by other so-called "deficits"—a tendency toward a firm commitment, toward perseverance, and toward loyalty and steadfastness.

Adults with Asperger Syndrome continue to be rule-oriented. This can apply to relationships in positive and negative ways. On one hand, the rules say that your boyfriend is your boyfriend (or your spouse is your spouse), and therefore you are true and faithful to that person. "They will be dedicated and true to the person they are with," said Dania Jakel of the Asperger's Association of New England. "They're steady and devoted, because they know the rules."

Similarly, because people with Asperger Syndrome tend to avoid conversations that involve small talk and banter, they may come across as more solemn and less flirtatious than other adults. Some men will seek relationships or marriage with women from foreign countries, particularly those with traditional cultures.

Often, adults with Asperger Syndrome who marry, or are in a committed partnership, improve notably in their social skills. And those deficits that remain are often more easily concealed, or they are compensated for by the spouse.

Community and Citizenship

The same factors that make adults with Asperger Syndrome constant and devoted spouses can also make them fine, upright citizens. Sometimes, their devotion to insisting on what's right can make them take on noble causes and pursue them with dogged persistence (sometimes to excess—speaking at length at public meetings, or writing endless letters to the editor).

Rarely, it seems, are these adults involved with antisocial or criminal behavior. They are far more likely to be victims than perpetrators. The exception, as with most behavior issues, is when they are misunderstood or make social blunders that offend or frighten others. Sometimes, a particular interest can become obsessive, with unfortunate results. One young man was imprisoned after being arrested for an unusual crime: stealing subway trains. He has been jailed nineteen times for transit-related crimes in and around New York, including taking the controls of a city bus, and dressing as a transit worker in order to enter the control room of a train station. Although this man has not been diagnosed, those who know him and know of his situation are quite certain that his obsessive behavior is an outgrowth of his Asperger Syndrome. They are working to get his case reevaluated in light of his disability.

Fortunately, cases like his are rare. Jerry Newport, who writes and lectures about Asperger Syndrome, described his adult life in remarks given before a conference on Asperger Syndrome. "I had, and still have, significant challenges, mainly in sensory areas. Where this hurt me the most is in vocational and social development, despite having unusual skills in memory and numerical calculation. You wouldn't expect someone who had several 800s on SAT tests and a national high school math award to wind up driving a taxi for over a decade...I can do many things well, if I don't have to think of anything else, but I am a lousy juggler, mentally and physically."

Despite his disability (or perhaps in part because of it), Newport has a unique and fascinating outlook on life. He sometimes describes Asperger Syndrome as "suburban autism." "My condition was maddeningly close to what most of my early peers...would have called 'eccentrically normal.' I had challenges, but mixed with enough normalcy to resemble growing up in the suburbs of autism."

Oftentimes, adults with Asperger Syndrome have adjusted so well, and have so successfully modified their stand-out behaviors, that—although they still have a lifelong disability—they do not appear disabled to casual observers.

You have, no doubt, met or worked with an adult with Asperger Syndrome without knowing it. They are members of the community, and many have successful lives, jobs, and marriages.

They still have difficulty figuring out "The Code." They still make social errors. They still have trouble coping with sensory overload, or being in chaotic settings. But they have, over the years, learned ways to manage, to seek out settings that work well, to buffer their sensitivities, to increase their skills and their flexibility, and to gain pride and self-esteem from their accomplishments.

And, in fact, those accomplishments are needed. We need human diversity. We need people with a rainbow of talents and abilities and outlooks. Fortunately for the rest of us, adults with Asperger Syndrome can proudly take their place in society and share their unique and remarkable perspectives with the world.

"The Letter I Never Wrote My Parents"

The following is a letter written by Jerry Newport, who is a founder of AGUA, a San Diego–based support and advocacy group for adults with autism and Asperger Syndrome. His poignant reflections reveal as no other description can the insights, the humor, the self-awareness—the full humanity—of people who are challenged in their social and communication abilities. As with so many people with Asperger Syndrome, Jerry has always found it difficult to express his emotions. And yet they were certainly there. His letter conveys the strong feelings he has about himself, his family, and specifically, his mother and father.

> Dear Mom and Dad,
>
> I paid you both a visit recently. You sure picked out a nice place to stretch out, though I am in no hurry to join you, you understand. Your cemetery is lovely, shared with an Indian Tribe in upper New York State. Just down the block is John

Newport, first Newport in America, at the corner, along with a
lot of other Newports; kind of a high rise plot. But your area is
by far the prettiest. Uncle Bob is still above ground, but his
headstone is already set up. Never accused you folks of last-
minute planning.

The occasion was Uncle Bob's 80th birthday. I think this is a
record for Newport males. At any rate, I represented our family.
John and Jim called in, but they have families in California, and
Jim could hardly walk off the set of "Fantasy Island" in Hawaii, to
attend any birthday party!

I got in the last word this time. I sat on a lovely marble
bench and blubbered out some news about how things have gone
in the years since the two of you reunited, in 1988. Dad, I guess
Mom got you caught up to what happened between 1969 and
then, but there have been some interesting recent events.

Guess what? I finally got married, and then, like John and
Jim, divorced. However, I learned much from the experience, and
having watched my older brothers become much happier in their
second marriages, hope the same happens to me someday. This is
just another example of what you did for me by having two sons
before me. Many of the things that did the most for me as a
child—baseball, scouting, band, etc.—were things that my brothers
did before me. They blazed the trail and it was easy to follow
because people expected me to do well if I was their younger
brother.

I'm really glad it turned out that way. I wonder what would
have happened if I had been born first. Would I have been so
frustrating that you would have thrown in the towel? I hope not,
by the way. John and Jim have turned out to be wonderfully
supportive adult brothers to each other and to me. They are
different, but have learned to respect those differences.

And what is that, you ask? What is it, whether it's me, or you
or my brothers, that makes a Newport a Newport? Just why do I
sit here, as I recently did at your resting place, nervously kneeling,

hovering over your headstone, finally shedding tears of gratitude that should have been shed in your living presence, but never were?

To be a Newport, I think, is to be a thoughtful, curious person with a deep sense of personal and public commitment. It is a struggle to balance this; all of the Newports I've met are pretty darn smart at something, if not many things, enough to feel adventurous or even irresponsibly drawn to a passion, be it art or math or whatever. But we also want to be with the community; we want our families, fireplaces, friends, pets and the trappings of the American Dream.

To be a Newport is often to be somewhat awkward, although in a lovable way. We are not usually major league athletic prospects, but we love our sports and outdoor pastimes. Indoors, we can turn a card table into our own IRA. We are not usually the life of the party but rarely miss one if invited. And we love to hear and tell long stories.

I know that both of you, on the last day of your lives, wondered what would become of me. The other brothers seemed on their way to their careers, John in public health and Jim in film production. But what of me? Your "math genius" seemed to have lost interest in math totally and had no interests at all to replace it. It was heartbreaking for both of you.

It was no picnic for me, either. None of us knew, as I grew up, that my occasional "Jerryisms," the way I could look askance and endlessly drone off on any subject, my extreme stage fright, my way of shutting down if I didn't have the absolute attention of the entire room, or my reputation for outlandish essays in the High School paper (the one on flatulence is still an Islip High School classic) were traits of a condition known as Asperger Syndrome.

Now, what does that mean? It means that some people are mostly normal and the part that isn't normal about them and may impede them from living to their fullest potential is explainable by behaviors that are common to Asperger Syndrome. People who are severely affected, exhibiting more frequent, intense and longer-lasting symptoms along with other problems (I wasn't) are known as autistic.

I have hesitated about using that word, autism, because both of you must have heard the myth about autism being caused by parents. Thankfully, that has been disproved and parents don't cause my much milder version, known as Asperger Syndrome, either.

What is more important is what you both taught all three of your sons: the value of ethics and discipline. The rewards of hard work. The importance of giving something back to the community. All of us carry on that tradition that you set every week, every time Dad did the accounting for our church or went out of his way to help an Islip High graduate find a job. Nor do we forget the countless unpaid hours Mom spent after school, helping a student. I am especially proud of what my older brothers have given back to the world.

John has been a great stepfather to five stepchildren. He has also been involved as a volunteer for numerous causes, even winding up in a *Newsweek* photo when he was part of an anti-fertility rite. He obviously has no dislike for children; he just thinks the world has enough of them already.

In 1984, Jim volunteered his talents to help design the course for the Olympic Equestrian Events in Fairbanks Ranch, San Diego County. In addition, although very successful in a highly competitive business, Jim has reached out, seen the good and personally rescued several friends who might not even be alive if he hadn't helped them through difficult times. His circle of friends has one thing in common: there is something in each one of them that Jim finds genuinely interesting. And they all share something else. They love Jimmy Newport because he is a Hollywood man with a heart.

There have been numerous times in my adulthood when I

was really out of hope. John and Jim always united to help me survive those times. I am very lucky to have the two older brothers you left me with. As for me, I have felt best when helping causes I believe in, whether it's whales, mass transit, or autism. I have given my time to lots of candidates, left and right. If there is a precinct in the city of San Diego that I haven't walked, it must be a new one. My proudest achievement was in 1978, when I led an effort to open up the city of San Diego to independent taxis and other forms of transit. The result has created thousands of small business opportunities and thousands of jobs. The *San Diego Reader* featured a photo of me in my custom-made "One Man, One Cab" T-shirt, in a centerfold with the other 49 top local newsmakers of 1978.

I am a late starter. I never could focus on more than one thing at a time. That's another trait often found in Asperger individuals. That worked out fine in high school. Everything was nicely scheduled and I did well. Once I got to college and was on my own, there were so many opportunities, academic, social and chemical, that I just got lost. I took drugs to blend in with the sixties crowd. Ironically, everyone else took them to get "screwed up." The intensity of the experience actually made me feel more normal! And since I could visually remember the details of each "trip," instant replays were cheap. In Ann Arbor, I was a very economical head.

It took two decades to get a sense of my self again, after I left Ann Arbor with a math degree and little interest in the field. It wasn't until a friend of mine told me to see a movie, *Rain Man,* that I began to understand why up to then, I felt so close to normal and so far away simultaneously. The movie was about a much more severely affected person than me, but his talent for numbers, like mine, was something that led me to find out more about people with autism.

I began reading about autism and felt lost for a couple of years. I just didn't feel, in comparison to autistic people, that I had ever had it so tough. I felt like I was something in between normal and autism, maybe a "mist-man," or an "aerosol man." Finally, I decided to go to an Autism Society meeting in 1991. That was a turning point. I met some adults more like me than I imagined and eventually learned about Asperger Syndrome.

Involvement with the autism community has rewarded me in ways I never expected. The local chapters helped me found my support group, which is now approaching its seventh anniversary. I have been abroad and to many places, to talk about adult issues with parents and professionals. It has given me the opportunity, for free, to learn from many experts.

A fellow board of directors member of ASA-LA, Dr. Linda Demer, helped me get a job at UCLA where at least sometimes, I get to use my natural ability with numbers. It is nice to work in the positive environment of a college campus. Of course, both of you must remember UCLA, as you were students there on sabbatical and saw Lew Alcindor, now known as Kareem Abdul-Jabbar, lead the Bruins to victory over Houston (109-69) and North Carolina (78-55) in the 1968 NCAA finals.

It is a lot easier to write now than a couple of pages ago. I guess when you are as emotionally constipated as I have been most of my 18,815 (and counting) days, it takes a lot of effort to finally risk sharing a feeling. But if anyone deserves to know that I feel something, especially something good about somebody, it's the two of you. Oh, remember all of those pets—the hamsters, dogs, cats, and parakeets we had? I still have pets and just recently helped my parakeets raise their first chick. She looks like her mother, Green Bean. I named her Brown-Eyed Girl.

I never said it enough when you were alive. I really miss the two of you now that my life is halfway sensible and I have things to share. But I want both of you to know, wherever your spirits have gone, that I and my older brothers all are, and will be, eternally grateful for what you did for us. We all love you and are proud to be your sons. I don't think I will be a parent, but I hope that when I leave this life someone will think that his life is better because I was a part of it. I learned that desire from the world's two best teachers, my parents.

I guess there isn't much left to say, except that I sure wish I had said a lot of this while you were still alive to hear it. But at least now you know that my love and appreciation were always there even if I had great difficulty expressing it. Thanks for being my parents. Nobody else could have done it any better.

Your youngest son,

Jerry Newport

11

Questions and Answers

Q: My husband and I are in dire need of respite. We both need to go out from time to time, but it's hard to find someone to babysit our eight-year-old daughter. Can we use a teenage babysitter without providing the sitter with a label? If I don't mention Asperger Syndrome, what should I tell her about our child?

A: It should be possible to leave your child with a capable older teenage sitter. It is essential to prepare any caregiver, but whether you use the actual diagnostic terminology is up to you. You will need to explain that your child has a learning disability that makes it difficult for her to understand language and facial expressions and so on. Give specific instructions on how to talk and play with her.

Likewise, prepare your child as well. Start out with a short session—perhaps hire the sitter to come for a brief session while you are still there, so you can be available to handle difficulties as they come up. Then you can go out for short periods, lengthening them as your child and the sitter grow better accustomed to one another.

Q: I'm worried my other child will think, every time he has a problem with anxiety or social skills, that maybe he has Asperger Syndrome, too. What can I say to reassure him?

A: Reassure your typical child that Asperger Syndrome is a neurological condition that you don't "catch" from someone else. Point out that some of their problems are not that much different from what everyone experiences from time to time—nervousness, worry, feeling confused or awkward in social situations, not understanding a joke, and so on. Explain that these normal experiences are part of life, and they have nothing to do with his brother's disorder. Point to specific things he can do, which his sibling cannot, that indicate his brain works in a typical way. Try to do this in a way that is respectful to the sibling with Asperger Syndrome.

Q: Will my child recognize if she is being bullied?

A: Not without help. This can be a real concern, because children with Asperger Syndrome can easily become victimized by other children who find them an easy mark. You will need to discuss this with your child, and talk about teasing and other unkind things kids do and say to one another. Remind her that all kids, not just those with Asperger Syndrome, suffer when they are teased or bullied, and that the bullies or teasers are breaking the rules. Encourage her to discuss teasing incidents with you. It may be better for you and your child to discuss the situation and decide together if it's serious.

Older children are more able to recognize unkind words and actions in others. In fact, they may misinterpret well-intentioned banter as unkindness or teasing, and respond inappropriately. Again, continue to discuss social difficulties with your child and brainstorm ways of responding.

Q: How strict should I be about my child remembering to do his homework? Is it fair to expect him to be responsible?

A: Homework is a difficult issue. Some children can, and should, be expected to accomplish their school work with reasonable support; others simply can't cope. This is an issue to discuss with your child's teacher and support staff at school. If your child really is unable to manage independent work at home, this can be included in his IEP as an accommodation. However, the *process* of homework (as the review, at home, of school work) is a good skill to build wherever possible. Ultimately, homework is about responsibility. And responsibility is a foundation skill for adulthood.

Q: My child does tend to rock repeatedly, which doesn't upset most people, but sometimes other children notice it and ask, "Hey. How come you're doing that?" What can I tell that child, and what should my child say?

A: See the discussion of disclosure in chapter 3. How you handle such questions depends on what you and your family have decided about how you want to present your child's disability to others. Often for young children, you can state simply, "Joan gets nervous sometimes in group situations like this party. She finds that rocking like that calms her down."

Or you can say, "Joan has a disability that makes her feel nervous when she's in a new situation. She feels calmer and more able to concentrate when she rocks." It's best to describe the disability functionally—that is, relate it to what she does and needs, rather than to terms and labels. Also, you can relate the disability to minor ones that most kids understand, such as wearing glasses, for example: sometimes parts of us don't work the way most people do and so we make adjustments to live our lives.

As you describe your child to others in her presence, and do so calmly and respectfully, you will be modeling ways that she can describe herself to others. But you should still teach her explicit ways to describe herself, and be sure to include her input and opinions about this. She may prefer the accurate diagnostic term, or may prefer to describe her challenge by saying, "I have a learning disability that makes it hard for me to figure out what people mean. That's why I get help with that in the Resource Room."

Q: In our family, we have always tried to teach our children how to manage money by giving each of them an allowance when they were old enough to make decisions about spending and saving. Our older kids caught on pretty well, learning how to make their money last and save for things they wanted. Our eight-year-old has Asperger Syndrome, and we are struck by how oddly he handles money. He has an allowance, but he never spends it. He accumulates the dollar bills and the coins and plays with them, arranging them and piling up the coins. He never thinks about money as something he can use to get something else he wants. How can we teach him some basic money skills as he grows older?

A: It's important to teach your child about the uses of money as part of personal responsibility and future independence. Most children with Asperger Syndrome have no difficulty learning coin and currency values as young children, and are usually quite capable of making arithmetic calculations. Later, you will need to teach specifically the important lessons of handling money: saving, budgeting, cost comparisons, and so on. For example, if he asks you to buy him something, you can tell him that that's what his money is for. Your son's obsessive approach to money and the currency itself is not a major concern. If he does have trouble later, it will be in the aspect of money management that involves organization and planning. The more he learns in childhood, the better able he'll be to cope later.

Q: What value, if any, does participating in theater or drama have for a student with Asperger Syndrome? My daughter is considering taking theater in tenth grade. She thinks she'll be able to meet boys, for one thing, and figures she will do well because she has an excellent memory and will have no trouble learning her lines. I'm concerned that she may find the experience overwhelming and become frustrated. Is this a good idea?

A: It can be a marvelous activity for a student with Asperger Syndrome who is eager to give it a try. Your child will probably do better acting in plays with traditional scripts, rather than in improvisational or comedy routines. The script and stage directions will offer comforting guidelines on what she should say, when and how to say it, and where to stand, sit, and so on. And the rehearsals will provide the kind of drill and practice that lend support and reassurance for kids with Asperger Syndrome. And even if she doesn't choose an acting role, there are many behind-the-scenes activities in any theatrical production to which she can apply her talents. Along with all of this there's the opportunity for socializing and friendship that comes with being part of a theater community. And in many schools, the theater "group" is more accepting of differences and eccentricity than others.

Q: Our older son is begging for a pet. He has his heart set on a golden retriever. But our younger son, who has Asperger Syndrome, is upset by anything that isn't predictable. Would he get used to a puppy? Or is there a better kind of pet for a family where a child has Asperger Syndrome?

A: The issue of pets is certainly a personal one. An anxious child may be upset by a large, smelly, rambunctious dog. Dogs tend to initiate play and interaction, whether their people are in the mood or not. Some children seem to feel more comfortable with cats, because, unlike dogs, they are more likely to give their humans a reasonable amount of space. Other children respond very well to horses.

But there's another point to consider here: is it fair to your older son to deny him the pleasure and learning experience of a dog? It might be better for everyone to work on ways to prepare your younger son, and perhaps minimize the puppy's impact on him. Perhaps his room could be off-limits, or the puppy could be restricted to a kennel cage during part of the day. By looking for ways to compromise and make reasonable accommodations, you should find a way to allow your older child his dog, and allow your younger child to maintain a comfort zone. Eventually, you may find that he grows quite attached to the dog.

Q: Our daughter is particularly sensitive to noises, especially the kind of vibrating buzzing sound given off by alarm clocks and the buzzer entries to buildings. She covers her ears and complains that it hurts her ears. She dislikes trips to the dentist, even though the dentist is very good with children, because of the unfamiliarity of the sensations, and the buzzing sound of the instrument the dentist uses to polish her teeth. At the last visit, he found a cavity, and we've scheduled an appointment to have it filled. I can't imagine how she will handle the sound and vibrations of the drill. Any suggestions to help her?

A: First, you are wise to take her to a dentist who is sensitive to children or anxious patients. Many pediatric dentists are real experts at reducing fear and anxiety in their patients. She may also be helped by a "dry run" of the procedure beforehand, including mock injections and drilling. The sound and sensation of the drill can indeed be very upsetting, and a good approach is to provide both masking sensations and competing sensations while this is going on. Thus, headphones with her preferred music or an interesting story tape can help. Beyond that, try to schedule the procedure as soon as possible, to minimize the buildup of worry, and see if it can be scheduled for the first or last time slot of the day, to minimize waiting.

Q: Our child is, as you can imagine, very upset when his routines or surroundings are changed. We have just learned that my company is relocating me to another city. It's a great opportunity, but we all have some concerns about leaving our familiar community and moving to an entirely new one. Our son, in particular, is upset. How can we help him cope with such a major upset in his life?

A: As with any major change in your child's life, preparation is the key. As soon as you know where you will live, what his room will look like, and something about his school, begin the process of describing his new routine. If he is young, focus on what his home life will be like, and emphasize the things that won't change—his familiar belongings, the household furniture, the pets, and, of course, your presence and love. Older children often enjoy doing research on the new community and may enjoy poring over maps of the new city. Try to involve the child in some aspect of planning for the move, so he becomes part of the team. In addition, an older child will need as much information as possible about his new school. No matter what, he will need considerable reassurance, and may ask questions repeatedly.

Q: We are expecting our second child in several months. How can we help our five-year-old adjust to all the changes that will take place in her life and her home?

A: All children benefit from preparation when they're about to have a new brother or sister. You can take the usual techniques for preparing typical kids, and apply or adapt them to your child's personality. You may avoid suggestions that are more oriented toward role-playing and symbolic elements (such as dolls and "new baby" children's books, for example), and focus on specific aspects of the household routine that will change, for better and for worse.

Prepare your five-year-old by talking about what is going to happen, involving her in the preparations by giving her certain responsibilities. She might choose a toy that she thinks the baby might like, or put baby clothes in the layette, or help arrange furniture in the baby's room.

Prepare, also, for her mother's absence. Naturally, when you go to the hospital, your child's routine will be very much changed. Prepare her specifically about that period of time: who will stay with her, where the hospital is, and when you are likely to return. She's old enough to understand the essentials of birth, and understand why you need to be at the hospital for a few days. Most hospitals give tours of the maternity unit specially designed for siblings-to-be.

After the baby arrives, try to schedule special one-on-one time with mother, father, grandparents, so that even though her familiar routines have been changed by the baby's arrival, she still feels the continuity of love and attachment from the family.

Some of the changes, naturally, will be difficult to adjust to—nighttime crying, tired parents, less time with parents, and so on. Others will be quite enjoyable, including a newfound sense of pride and accomplishment as your older child learns that she can do useful things for you and the baby and be rewarded for them.

Your younger child will change and bring new challenges as he develops, learns to walk and talk and get into his older sister's things. But those changes occur gradually in babies, and your older child will be able to adjust to all these variations in family routine as they occur.

Q: We've had the same nanny for all three of our children. She's been wonderful, and our youngest, who has Asperger Syndrome, has known her all his life. Now she is about to retire, and we're going to have to find a replacement. How can we help our son adjust to such a major change in his life?

A: Social Stories (see chapter 8) are useful tools in preparing children for the inevitable changes in life. Once you are sure what is going to happen—when the nanny will leave, and who the new one will be—have a Social Story that deals with the concept, "Things Change." Help your child understand what he liked about the person, and try to have that duplicated in the new person.

Keep in mind that new people may fill similar roles, and do some with some degree of consistency. Stress the consistency. Point out that one of the things he liked about the nanny, for example, was that she liked to tell the kids stories. Suggest that the new person also likes to tell stories, and she'll have some interesting new ones.

Have the child care person who is leaving make up an "owner's manual" for your child, explaining what works and what is less likely to work well with your child. This will provide a foundation for the training and preparation you will do with the new person.

Q: The other day I was stressed out myself, because of pressures at work and my kids getting my goat at home. When my daughter absolutely refused to get ready for her piano lesson, I just lost it, and screamed at her. Naturally that upset her, and she burst into tears and ran to her room. I apologized, but I'm not sure if I really explained it very well. What should I tell her about what happened that she can really understand and appreciate?

A: The best way to explain this kind of situation is to keep it simple, clear, and focused on rules. Avoid deep analysis of the why and hows. You can say, "I was feeling worried and distracted because of my own job. So when you refused to cooperate, I got upset. I yelled at you, and you got upset. I shouldn't have done what I did. I should have counted to ten, and then explained what I felt. I'm sorry, and I'll try to do better."

Notice that in describing things in this short, to-the-point way, you are actually modeling language she can use when she makes mistakes of her own. You are performing a Social Autopsy on your own behavior, saying, "This is what I did, this is the unfortunate effect it had, this is what I should have done and will try to do next time."

Finally, once it's been explained, put it behind you and move on.

Q: I know I should teach my son the "rules" in a specific, literal manner. But often when I attempt to do this, he resists and refuses and won't listen or comply. How do I accomplish this without his cooperation?

A: In some ways, that's one of the challenges that all children present. They don't always obey us, no matter how much we try to handle them the "right" way. With typical kids, you might just say, "OK, it's your funeral," and let them learn from the awful consequences of their bad behavior. With Asperger Syndrome, however, you can't count on that. It may take several sessions and repetitions before you see improvement.

The best thing to do is emphasize rules. If it's a really top-priority rule, you'll have to be very methodical and stubborn yourself. Tell your child, this is the rule. This is what you are expected to do. This is what will happen when you do it (good thing), and this is what will happen if you don't (bad thing). Be consistent. And, as always, find ways to reward your child when he does follow through with the expected behavior.

Q: My child with Asperger Syndrome needs far more supervision than my other child. Yet she points out that we impose different rules for her and for her sister, who is only a year older. Kate gets to stay out late, go places without us, travel on her own, and so on, but Laura cannot. Should I try to keep the rules the same for both, or if not, how would I explain this?

A: In any family, some of the rules and regulations are universal, and apply to everyone. Those might include saying grace before meals, or taking one's shoes off before entering the house. Other kinds of rules, however, have to be tailored to each person. That's the kind that Laura is concerned with here. In those situations, rules don't have to be "the same" in order to be "fair." People have different needs and abilities. It would be unfair for Kate to have the same restrictions Laura requires, and it wouldn't be safe for Laura to have the same freedoms that Kate enjoys. You can also explain that Laura will develop more responsibility as she grows older, and with that responsibility comes greater freedom.

Q: My son is attending a support group for kids with Asperger Syndrome. It seems like a good idea, but I have some concerns about his developing friendships with other kids with Asperger Syndrome. Should I be concerned that hanging out with other kids with the same disorder will make it harder for him to overcome his social difficulties? What would you suggest?

A: Support groups are an excellent resource for kids with Asperger Syndrome. Friendships do, indeed, develop within these groups, but their primary purpose is twofold: to provide kids with the emotional support that comes of getting together with others who truly understand their difficulties, and to provide an opportunity for companionship and socializing with a tolerant and understanding group. I wouldn't be too concerned about your son modeling inappropriate socializing as long he also has some opportunity to associate with typical kids as well. As he gets older, such a group can provide a real sanctuary from the more difficult emotional upheavals of adolescence.

Q: My brother and sister and I, and our families, have always gotten together for a week's vacation each summer. Recently, I've sensed that they are pulling away from the idea, and I'm thinking it may be because of my eight-year-old. She has recently been diagnosed with Asperger Syndrome, which explains her problems getting along with people. She alternately complains about everything, in an annoying way, or withdraws and refuses to participate. The others never know what to expect from her. I understand that they would rather have a peaceful time without our problems, but I'm hurt at the idea that they would want to exclude my child. What's the best thing to do for my daughter's best interests?

A: First, it would be wise to make sure that your intuition is accurate. You might approach the family member whom you consider the most sympathetic to your concerns, and ask calmly if they have concerns about going on the vacation, and if there is anything they would like you to do. If indeed the problem does seem to be in their responses to your child's behavior, you'll have to make some choices. If there are compromises you could make to make the occasion more pleasurable for all, consider that. For example, it may be that your relatives feel they don't know how to relate to your child, or talk to her, or discipline her. If that's the case, you might offer to stay with your daughter as much as possible, minimizing the time the other adults have to try to cope. Or you might offer to give the others a crash course in what works, and doesn't work, with your daughter. Or, if you sense that your family is unable to relate with understanding and kindness, you'll have to look out for your child's ultimate interests and consider foregoing the vacation.

Q: My son plays the trumpet and is interested in being in the marching band in high school. He is talented musically, but he's very shy, and he's not particularly well coordinated. Is this a good choice?

A: A lot depends on the individual. Being in a demanding, organized activity such as the band could be overwhelming for some kids with Asperger Syndrome, particularly those who would find the loud music upsetting or would become overly anxious. But the structure and routines that are inevitable in such activities might be ideal for a child who is musical and has expressed an interest. If he does join, prepare him by discussing what he might do if he forgets a marching step (watch the other kids, for example), or feels a panic attack coming (take breaths, use his relaxation techniques, for example). Also, be sure to discuss his participation with the adult musical director, and be sure that person is on board and aware of how to work best with your son.

The bonus, of course, is that if this does work, band provides your son with a group to belong to and socialize with. As always, the best way to forge friendship is through shared interests and activities, and this kind of group could be ideal for your son.

Q: We have always loved hiking, and would like to take a backpacking trip with our family. Our younger daughter has never enjoyed hiking, and now that we know she has Asperger Syndrome, we have a better understanding of what she didn't like about it: her feet always hurt, she hated the food, she wanted to go home, and so on. Is there a way that we can enjoy this activity as a family, and still include our daughter?

A: In a situation like this, compromise and preparation are key. You might begin by considering a trip that is perhaps less demanding than the expert hikers in the family might like, but within reach for your daughter. You could talk to her about what to expect, the accommodations you'll put into place to address her particular concerns, and your expectation that she meets you halfway.

You might allow her to wear her familiar beat-up sneakers, instead of proper hiking boots, if that's what she's comfortable with. You might also cut her some slack in other areas. You might take along more of her possessions than most backpackers would, for example—her pillow, a portable tape player, books. You could keep her backpack lighter than yours. She might have her own tent as a sanctuary, and have quiet time with her books while other members of the family take a challenging climb.

Once you've assured her that you'll try to keep her as comfortable as possible, try to involve her in planning the trip. She might study weather reports, map out the itinerary on an atlas, look up information on National Parks on the Internet, or calculate what foods and supplies need to be purchased and packed.

Ultimately, both she and the rest of you will benefit if you can all share this adventure. If you accommodate her particular needs without sacrificing the broader experience, everyone will benefit.

Q: Our teenage son has terrible, explosive rages. When he was little they were tantrums, but as he's grown older they are more threatening to others and I worry they'll get him into serious trouble. He screams, pounds tables, and throws things. What can we do to help him manage this anger?

A: When an episode occurs, the first priority is to get through it safely. Try to stay calm and de-escalate the situation. Do not try to have a discussion or analysis during the episode, because your son is unlikely to be able to absorb much useful information while he is so upset.

After things calm down, do try to determine what set him off. It may be a disappointment, wounded feelings, a surprise or disruption in his routine, or a sensory assault. It's important to identify the cause in order to prevent a recurrence.

Armed with this information, you and he can conduct a Social Autopsy and perhaps work on Social Stories to follow when he feels anger coming on.

Bear in mind that being out of control is a highly unpleasant sensation for someone with Asperger Syndrome. Your son is not lashing out because he enjoys it, but because he is unable to contain his stress.

If he hurts himself or others, or places people or property at risk, you'll need to take this a step farther and seek professional help, which may include anger management techniques or medication.

Q: My daughter is fourteen, and very naive. I'm concerned about how I can protect her from being exploited. She's very intelligent, but lacks common sense. What should I do?

A: Your child does run a greater risk than other teenagers, so she will probably need more supervision than others. You will need to strike a balance between keeping her safe and under your watchful eye, and giving her opportunities to learn about the ways of the world.

You will have to teach her explicitly and specifically what dangers she might come across, along with ways of dealing with them. These would include Social Stories, scripts, and "What-if?" sessions. In particular, emphasize sexual safety, and the "rule" that her body is her own property, and she has the right to say "no."

As you do this, try to avoid sensationalizing the dangers that concern you so much that you increase her anxiety. Be matter-of-fact in tone, rather than gee-whiz, as you and she work on issues of safety and independence. Reassure her that she can learn to handle herself in many situations as long as she takes her time and keeps communication open with you.

Q: How do I keep our family life hyperorganized? I know that's best for kids with Asperger Syndrome, but it's tough enough for families these days, and I myself am not the most organized or efficient person in the world (I may have some of those Executive Function shortfalls myself).

A: Get books from the library about household organization and apply them with a grain of salt. Many are difficult to follow consistently, but there may be some tips about organizing your home and your schedule that will work in your family.

Concentrate on those areas that directly affect your child and his sense of order and security. Schedules, in particular, are often of great importance to children with Asperger Syndrome, so calendars and lists will not only help establish order in your household, but provide visual reassurance for your child. You might use a large, business-style calendar with plenty of room to note activities and appointments. Or you might keep two calendars, using one exclusively for your child's activities.

Make organizing your child's routine and schedule the top priority. There's no harm done if your own closet is a mess, or your garage disorganized, as long as your child's life has order and structure in it.

Q: My husband and I are separating. How should we handle the custody of our daughter, who has Asperger Syndrome?

A: Divorce is never an easy situation for children, but you can make the best of it with as much consistency as possible. Children with Asperger Syndrome, like all children, very much need to know that both parents love them and want them. You'll have to work harder than other parents to coordinate household routines so that your child feels safe and comfortable in both households.

Your child will take visitation schedules very seriously, both because they are predictable and because they are "the rule." Make sure to adhere to the schedule closely. If a change can't be avoided, prepare your child as much as possible. Pre-teach, plan, and predict changes in advance. Structure and predictability help smooth most transitions, and even a major one like this can be managed.

Finally, whatever your relationship with your daughter's father, allow your child to have "an oasis of agreement" within that relationship. In other words, you may disagree on many things with your ex-spouse, but you can come together to make sure her needs are met.

Q: What kinds of punishments or negative consequences would work best with our son? Obviously spanking is out, but what can we try that will be negative, but not so upsetting that it defeats the purposes?

A: Much depends on your child's age, and on the type of misbehavior in question. First and foremost, remember that the most important consequences are positive ones, where you "catch your child doing the *right* thing." These consequences are educative, and promote positive behavior by acknowledging positive behavior.

Removal of cherished privileges also has an impact, especially if it involves separation from the child's area of special interest. A very young child with a passion for Thomas the Tank Engine, for example, could have his time with his favorite toy restricted as a consequence for misbehavior.

Time-outs may work if your child's misbehavior seems to stem from either stress or inappropriate attention-seeking. They may not be appropriate if your child has a tendency to spend too much time alone or withdraw into a shell, or if his misbehavior seems intentionally designed to avoid doing something.

Ignoring is sometimes a better approach for behavior that seems designed to provoke attention.

Consequences need to be negative in the sense that they should not reinforce inappropriate behavior, but they should not be hurtful or shaming in any way.

Q: My fourteen-year-old child refuses to spend time socially. She spends all her time in her room. When we try to encourage her to go out, she says the other kids are "stupid" and "boring." She refuses to attend a support group. What should we do?

A: Recognize that she may be more comfortable alone. Many kids with Asperger Syndrome need a lot more solitary time than other kids. You'll have to help her strike a balance between the solitude she's comfortable with and the opportunity to develop social skills. It's best to compromise, negotiate, and then agree upon specific rules about how much time she will spend alone, and what efforts she will make to reach out. Consider her area of interest as a "hook" to create outside interests and social opportunities.

Q: My child's teacher bristles when I try to tell her how to teach someone with Asperger Syndrome. She's a good teacher for my child, but doesn't want me to tell her how to teach and seems dismissive of my suggestions. What should I do?

A: It would be a good idea to find out what is behind her attitude. Is she overwhelmed by too many students with too many different needs? Do your suggestions involve too much preparation time? Is she getting insufficient help from support staff? Is she interpreting your suggestions as micromanaging her technique?

Ultimately, you have the right and responsibility to be closely involved in your child's educational experience. Your child's Individual Education Plan (IEP) is a legal document, and the teacher is obligated to follow it. Seek out help from other members of your child's IEP team, tactfully if possible, but persistently. Insist on your child's legal rights, and the correct application of the IEP.

Q: My child was playing with a neighbor child and the two were starting to roughhouse in the back yard. At one point, my son took a shovel and hit the other child on the back, really hard. He didn't seem the least bit sorry. Is it that he has trouble with empathy, or is he just plain mean?

A: Sometimes children and adults with Asperger Syndrome can seem remarkably insensitive to the feelings of others. But the chances are that your son was not intentionally trying to hurt the other child. He may have misinterpreted the horsing around that was going on, and lashed out. Or, he might have played out a scene he saw in a cartoon (*Roadrunner* cartoons are notorious for these). Either way, he demonstrated poor critical thinking skills, and a lack of judgment about the situation.

Unless this is an isolated incident, you'll certainly want to keep an eye on the play activities in your yard, since the safety of all concerned is an issue. But from your son's standpoint, the best bet is to treat the offense like another social faux pas. Review, explain in concrete terms what happened, and what course of action might have been better. Create a Social Story. And it would be a good idea for your son to apologize, which is always appropriate when we've hurt or offended others. He might do this by letter if it's difficult for him to do it face-to-face.

Q: How do people with Asperger Syndrome handle their spiritual dimension? Are they able to experience and appreciate religious and spiritual things? Do they join churches or religious communities?

A: As with all aspects of adults with Asperger Syndrome, it's necessary to be somewhat speculative, since so few now-adults were diagnosed as children. Most likely, they are similar to the typical population: some are essentially nonreligious, others are devout, with a whole continuum in between. What we do know from what adults have told us is that while they may be less enthusiastic about some of the metaphorical aspects of organized religion, they often respond well to beauty in a spiritual way, as they do with music, art, and natural wonders. Some adults find great comfort in religions that are essentially rule-oriented, such as fundamentalist denominations, or sects in which rules of conduct are laid out plainly, are expected to be followed, and in which people who follow them are admired and respected.

Q: What kind of parent might my child with Asperger Syndrome hope to become as an adult?

A: Again, we don't know a great deal, other than anecdotally, about adults with Asperger Syndrome. Although marriage and children may be less common, they certainly occur. We would expect the whole range of parenting experiences and abilities that we find in the "typical" community. There's no reason that adults with Asperger Syndrome couldn't be capable parents, especially if they have learned ways of managing their difficulties, and have structured a supportive and nurturing life.

Resources

Internet Sources and Organizations

OASIS (Online Asperger Syndrome
   Information and Support)
www.aspergersyndrome.org
The OASIS Web site, organized by
   Barbara Kirby, provides an excellent
   entry into up-to-date information
   about Asperger Syndrome and is an
   excellent way to get in touch with
   current support groups.

Other useful Internet sites include:

ASPEN, INC. (Asperger Syndrome
   Education Network)
www.aspennj.org/
A New Jersey–based education, support,
   and advocacy organization.

ASC-US
P.O. Box 49267
Jacksonville Beach, FL 32240-9267
(904) 745-6741
www.asc-us.org
The national organization providing
   information, support, and advocacy
   for families of individuals with
   Asperger Syndrome.

National Institute of Neurological
   Disorders and Stroke (NINDS)
   Asperger Syndrome Information
   Page
www.ninds.nih.gov/health_and_medical/
   disorders/asperger_doc.htm
This government site provides

information on the latest research and treatment related to neurological disorders, including Asperger Syndrome.

The Autism Society of America
7910 Woodmont Ave., Suite 300
Bethesda, MD 20814-3067
(301) 657-0881
(800) 3-AUTISM
www.autism-society.org
Advocates for individuals with autism spectrum disorders and their families, and provides information including conferences and a newsletter.

Tony Attwood, who has written extensively on Asperger Syndrome, has a Web site with up-to-date information.
www.tonyattwood.com

Learning Disability Association of America (LDA)
4156 Library Road
Pittsburgh, PA 15234-1349
(412) 341-1515
www.ldanatl.org
A national support organization for those with learning disabilities and their families. Provides information, advocacy, and referrals to over 500 affiliates.

Maap Services
P.O. Box 524
Crown Point, IN 46308
(219) 662-1311
www.maapservices.org
Maap is an exceptional organization that serves people with autism, Asperger Syndrome, and PDD:NOS and those who are family members and caregivers. Their quarterly newsletter, *The Maap,* is circulated in 47 countries.

National Information Center for Children and Youth with Disabilities (NICHCY)
P.O. Box 1492
Washington, DC 20013-1492
(800) 695-0285
www.nichcy.org
A governmental organization that can provide resources to parents on agencies and organizations involved with any disability. Maintains a "State Resource Sheet" with valuable contacts.

NLD on the Web
www.nldontheweb.org
This is an excellent Web site for information and resources relating to Nonverbal Learning Disability. It contains references, articles, and important links to the NLD community.

Software and Technology

Closing the Gap
P.O. Box 68
526 Main St.
Henderson, MN 56044
(507) 248-3294
www.closingthegap.com
Information and sources for computer
   technology for persons with
   disabilities.

Superduperinc.com
(800) 277-8737
Books and games for use by speech and
   language pathologists, special
   education teachers, and parents.

Alphasmart Inc.
20400 Stevens Creek Blvd., Suite 300
Cupertino, CA 95014
www.alphasmart.com
Keyboarding systems for children with
   dysgraphia.

State and Local Resources

The following listing includes public
   agencies that provide educational,
   vocational, and advocacy services to
   people with developmental disabilities.
   For information on local organizations
   and support groups, consult the
Autism Society of America Web site
and the OASIS Web site.

Alabama

AL Department of Education, Division
   of Special Education Services
P.O. Box 302101
Montgomery, AL 36130-2101
(334) 242-8114
(800) 392-8020 (in AL)
www.alsde.edu/speced/speced.html

Special Needs Programs, Department of
   Education
Gordon Persons Building
P.O. Box 302101
Montgomery, AL 36130-2101
(334) 242-9108

Alabama Developmental Disabilities
   Planning Council
RSA Union Building
100 N. Union St.
P.O. Box 301410
Montgomery, AL 36130-1410
(334) 242-3973, (800) 232-2158

Alabama Disabilities Advocacy Program
   (ADAP)
P.O. Box 870395
Tuscaloosa, AL 35487
(205) 348-4928, (800) 826-1675
www.adap.net

Children's Rehabilitation Service
Alabama Department of Rehabilitation
  Services
2129 E. South Blvd.
P.O. Box 11586
Montgomery, AL 36111-0586
(334) 281-8780, (800) 846-3697
www.rehab.state.al.us

Autism Society of Alabama
771 Second St.
Helena, AL 35080
(205) 621-0548
(877) 428-8476 (toll-free)
www.autism-alabama.org

Alaska
Office of Special Education
Alaska Department of Education
801 W. 10th St., Suite 200
Juneau, AK 99801-1894
(907) 465-8702
www.educ.state.ak.us/tls/sped

State of Alaska Department of Health &
  Social Services
Special Needs Services Unit
1231 Gambell St.
Anchorage, AK 99501-4627
(907) 269-3460

Division of Vocational Rehabilitation
801 W. 10th St., M.S. 0581
Juneau, AK 99801
(907) 269-3573

Disability Law Center of Alaska
615 E. 82nd, Suite 1101
Anchorage, AK 99518
(907) 344-1002

American Samoa
Special Education Division
Department of Education
Pago Pago, AS 96799
(684) 633-1323

Department of Human & Social Services
Division of Vocational Rehabilitation
Pago Pago, AS 96799
(684) 699-1371

AS Developmental Disabilities Council
P.O. Box 194
Pago Pago, AS 96799
(684) 633-5908

Protection and Advocacy for Developmental Disabilities
Office of Protection and Advocacy for
  the Disabled
P.O. Box 3937
Pago Pago, AS 96799
(684) 633-2441

Arizona

Exceptional Student Services
Department of Special Education
1535 West Jefferson
Phoenix, AZ 85007
(602) 542-4013
www.ade.state.az.us

Rehabilitation Services Bureau 930A
Department of Economic Security
1789 W. Jefferson 2NW
Phoenix, AZ 85007
(602) 542-3332

Arizona Center for Disability Law
3839 N. 3rd St. #209
Phoenix, AZ 85012
(602) 274-6287
www.acdl.com

Arkansas

Special Education Unit, Department of
   Education
State Education Building C,
   Room 105
#4 Capitol Mall
Little Rock, AR 72201-1071
(501) 682-4225

Department of Workforce Education
Arkansas Rehabilitation Services
1616 Brookwood Drive
P.O. Box 3781
Little Rock, AR 72203-3781
(501) 296-1616

Disability Rights Center
1100 N. University,
Suite 201
Little Rock, AR 72207
(501) 296-1775
(800) 482-1174
www.advocacyservices.org

California

Special Education, Department of
   Education
P.O. Box 944272
Sacramento, CA 94244-2720
(916) 445-4613
www.cde.ca.gov/spbranch/sed/index.htm

State Council on Developmental
   Disabilities
2000 O St., Room 100
Sacramento, CA 95814
(916) 322-8481

Center for Autism and Related Disorders
23300 Ventura Blvd.
Woodland Hills, CA 91364
(818) 223-0123

Autism Society of California
P.O. Box 1295
Escondido, CA 92033
(800) 700-0037

Colorado

Special Education Services Unit/
   Colorado Dept. of Education
201 E. Colfax Ave.
Denver, CO 80203
(303) 866-6694

Division of Vocational Rehabilitation
Department of Human Services
110 16th St., 2nd Floor
Denver, CO 80202
(303) 620-4153

Colorado Developmental Disabilities
   Planning Council
777 Grant St., Suite 304
Denver, CO 80203
(303) 894-2345

The Legal Center for People with
   Disabilities and Older People
455 Sherman St., Suite 130
Denver, CO 80203-4403
(303) 722-0300
(800) 288-1376 (in CO)
www.thelegalcenter.org

Connecticut

Bureau of Special Education & Pupil
   Services
CT Dept. of Education
25 Industrial Park Road
Middletown, CT 06457-1520
(860) 807-2025

Council on Developmental Disabilities
160 Capitol Ave.
Hartford, CT 06120-1308
(860) 418-6160

Autism Society of Connecticut
125 Harrington St.
Meriden, CT 06451
(203) 235-7629
www.geocities.com/HotSprings/Spa/7896

The Center for Children with Special
   Needs
384Z Merrow Road
Tolland, CT 06084
(860) 870-5313
Michael D. Powers, Psy.D., Director
Provides diagnostic, evaluation,
   consultation, and treatment services
   for individuals with Asperger
   Syndrome, autism, and related
   PDDs.

Connecticut Autism Spectrum Resource
   Center
300 East Rock Rd.
New Haven, CT 06511
(203) 787-3676
www.ct-asrc.org
CTASRC provides families in
   Connecticut with a range of
   important services, including updated
   information, referrals, advocacy, and
   professional development sessions
   for parents and professionals alike.

Through its goal of active empowerment of families, the Center fills an essential need for families.

Yale Child Study Center
Yale University School of Medicine
230 South Frontage Road
P.O. Box 207900
New Haven, CT 06520-7900
(203) 785-2510
www.yale.edu/chldstdy/autism/index.
html
Provides diagnostic, evaluation, and treatment services for individuals with Asperger Syndrome and other PDDs. A leading center of research on Asperger Syndrome in the United States.

Delaware
Exceptional Children and Early Childhood Group
Department of Education
P.O. Box 1402
Dover, DE 19903-1402
(302) 739-4667
www.doe.state.de.us

Delaware Division of Vocational Rehabilitation
4425 N. Market St.
P.O. Box 9969
Wilmington, DE 19809-0969
(302) 761-8275

Delaware Developmental Disabilities Council
Margaret M. O'Neill Bldg., 2nd Floor
410 Federal St., Suite 2
Dover, DE 19901
(302) 739-3333
www.state.de.us/ddc

Autism Society of Delaware
P.O. Box 7336
Wilmington, DE 19803-0336
(302) 777-7273
www.wserv.com/delautism

District of Columbia
Rehabilitation Services Administration
Department of Health and Human Services
810 First St., NE, 10th Floor
Washington, DC 20002
(202) 442-8663

DC Developmental Disabilities State Planning Council
2700 Martin L. King, Jr. Ave., SE
Department of Human Services
801 East Building
Washington, DC 20032
(202) 279-6086

Florida

Bureau of Instructional Support and
Community Services
Division of Public Schools and
Community Education
Department of Education
325 W. Gaines St., Suite 614
Tallahassee, FL 32399-0400
(850) 488-1570

Division of Vocational Rehabilitation
Department of Labor and Employment
Security
2002 Old St. Augustine Road, Building A
Tallahassee, FL 32399-0696

Florida Developmental Disabilities Council
124 Marriott Drive, Suite 203
Tallahassee, FL 32301-2981
(850) 488-4180

Autism Society of Florida, Inc.
2858 Remington Green Circle
Tallahassee, FL 32308
(850) 997-7233

Georgia

Division for Exceptional Students
GA Department of Education
1870 Twin Towers East
Atlanta, GA 30334
(404) 656-3963
www.doe.k12.ga.us/sla/exceptional/
exceptional.asp

Department of Human Resources
Division of Rehabilitation Services
2 Peachtree St., NW, 35th Floor
Atlanta, GA 30303-3142
(404) 657-3000
www.vocrehabga.org

Governor's Council on Developmental
Disabilities
2 Peachtree St., NW, 3rd Floor,
Suite 210
Atlanta, GA 30303-3142
(404) 657-2126
(888) 275-4233
www.ga-ddcouncil.org

Greater Georgia Chapter
Autism Society of America
2971 Flowers Road, South, Suite 140
Atlanta, GA 30341
(770) 451-0954
www.asaga.com

Guam

Special Education Division
GU Department of Education
P.O. Box DE
Hagatna, GU 96932
(671) 475-0552

GU Developmental Disabilities Council
104 E. St.
Tiyan, GU 96913
(671) 475-9127

GLSC Disability Law Center Services
113 Bradley Place
Hagatna, GU 96910
(671) 477-9811

Hawaii
Special Education Section
Hawaii Department of Education
637 18th Ave., Room 102
Honolulu, HI 96816
(808) 733-4990
www.doe.k12.hi.us

Division of Vocational Rehabilitation
Department of Human Services
601 Kamokila Blvd., Room 515
Kapolei, HI 96707
(808) 586-5355

Protection and Advocacy Agency
1580 Makaloa St., Suite 1060
900 Fort Street Mall, Suite 1040
Honolulu, HI 96813
(808) 949-2922
(800) 882-1057 (in HI)
www.pixi.com/pahi

Autism Society of Hawaii
P.O. Box 2995
Honolulu, HI 96802
(808) 256-7540

Idaho
Bureau of Special Education Section
Idaho Department of Education
P.O. Box 83720
Boise, ID 83720-0027
(208) 332-6910

Division of Vocational Rehabilitation
P.O. Box 83720
Boise, ID 83720-0096
(208) 334-3390

Autism Society of America—Treasure
Valley Chapter
2811 East Migratory Drive
Boise, ID 83706

Illinois
Office of Rehabilitation Services
Department of Human Services
P.O. Box 19429
Springfield, IL 62794-9429
(217) 524-3824

Illinois Planning Council on Developmental Disabilities
830 S. Spring St.
Springfield, IL 62704
(217) 782-9696

Autism Society of Illinois
2200 S. Main St., Suite 317
Lombard, IL 60148
(708) 691-1270

Indiana
Division of Special Education
Department of Education
State House, Room 229
Indianapolis, IN 46204-2798
(317) 232-0570

Indiana Family and Social Services
    Administration
Vocational Rehabilitation Services
Division of Disability, Aging and
    Rehabilitative Services
402 W. Washington St., Room W453
P.O. Box 7083
Indianapolis, IN 46207-7083
(317) 232-1319
(800) 545-7763, ext. 1319

Indiana Resource Center for Autism
2853 E. Tenth St.
Bloomington, IN 47408-2696
(812) 855-6508
www.isdd.indiana.edu/~irca

Iowa
Bureau of Family and Community Services
Department of Education
Grimes State Office Building
Des Moines, IA 50319-0146
(515) 281-5735
www.state.ia.us/educate/index/html

Governor's Developmental Disabilities
    Council
617 E. Second St.
Des Moines, IA 50309
(515) 281-9083

Autism Society of Iowa
3135 Spring Valley Road
Dubuque, IA 52001
(319) 557-1169

Kansas
Student Support Services
Kansas State Department of Education
120 E. 10th Ave.
Topeka, KS 66612
(785) 291-3097

Developmental Disabilities Services
SRS/MH & Developmental Disabilities
Docking State Office Building,
    5th Floor North
Topeka, KS 66612-1570
(785) 296-3561

Kansas Autism Foundation (KAF)
1605 Vermont Ave.
Lawrence, KS 66044

Kentucky

Division of Exceptional Children's
Services
Kentucky Department of Education
Capitol Plaza Tower, 8th Floor
500 Mero St.
Frankfort, KY 40601
(502) 564-4970
www.kde.state.ky.us

Department of Vocational
Rehabilitation
Cabinet for Workforce Development
209 St. Clair
Frankfort, KY 40601
(502) 564-4440

Kentucky Developmental Disabilities
Planning Council
100 Fair Oaks Lane, 4E-F
Frankfort, KY 40621-0001
(502) 564-7842

Department for Public Advocacy,
P&A Division
100 Fair Oaks Lane, 3rd Floor
Frankfort, KY 40601
(502) 564-2967
(800) 372-2988 (in KY)

Louisiana

Division of Special Populations
Louisiana State Department of
Education
P.O. Box 94064
Baton Rouge, LA 70804-9064
(225) 342-3633

Department of Social Services/LA
Rehabilitation Services
8225 Florida Blvd.
Baton Rouge, LA 70806-4834
(225) 925-4131

LA State Planning Council on
Developmental Disabilities
P.O. Box 3455
Baton Rouge, LA 70821-3455
(225) 342-6804
(800) 922-3425 (in LA)
www.laddc.org

Maine

Department of Education, Office of
Special Services
23 State House Station
Augusta, ME 04333-0023
(207) 287-5950; (207) 287-2550
www.state.me.us/education/speced

Bureau of Rehabilitation Services
Department of Labor
150 State House Station
Augusta, ME 04333
(207) 287-5100

ME Developmental Disabilities Council
139 State House Station, Nash Building
Capitol and Sewall Streets
Augusta, ME 04333-0139
(207) 287-4213
(800) 244-3990 (in ME)

Autism Society of America
693 Western Ave., Suite 2
Manchester, ME 04351
(207) 626-2708
(800) 273-5200 (in ME)

Maryland

Department of Education, Division of
    Special Education
Early Intervention Services
200 W. Baltimore St.
Baltimore, MD 21201-2595
(410) 767-0238
www.msde.state.md.us

Division of Rehabilitation Services
Department of Education
Maryland Rehabilitation Center
2301 Argonne Drive
Baltimore, MD 21218-1696
(410) 554-9385
www.dors.state.md.us/

Maryland Developmental Disabilities
    Council
300 West Lexington St., Box 10
Baltimore, MD 21201-2323
(410) 333-3688

Maryland Disability Law Center
1800 N. Charles, Suite 204
Baltimore, MD 21201
(410) 727-6352
(800) 233-7201

Massachusetts

Educational Improvement Group
Department of Education
350 Main St.
Malden, MA 02148-5023
(781) 338-3000
www.doe.mass.edu

Massachusetts Rehabilitation
    Commission
Fort Point Place
27-43 Wormwood St.
Boston, MA 02210-1616
(617) 204-3600

Massachusetts Developmental
    Disabilities Council
174 Portland St., 5th Floor
Boston, MA 02114
(617) 727-6374
Disability Law Center, Inc.
11 Beacon St., Suite 925
Boston, MA 02108
(617) 723-8455
(800) 872-9992
www.dlc-ma.org

Community Resources for People with
Autism
116 Pleasant Place
Easthampton, MA 01027
(413) 529-2428
www.crocker.com/~crautism

Asperger's Association of New England
(AANE)
1301 Centre St.
Newton Centre, MA 02459
(617) 527-2894
www.aane.org

Michigan
Office of Special Education and Early
Intervention Services
Department of Education
608 W. Allegan St.
Lansing, MI 48933
(517) 373-9433
www.mde.state.mi.us/off/sped

Michigan Department of Career Devel-
opment
Michigan Rehabilitation Services
P.O. Box 30010
Lansing, MI 48909
(517) 373-3391

Michigan Developmental Disabilities
Council
Lewis Cass Building
Lansing, MI 48913
(517) 334-6123

Michigan Protection and Advocacy Service
106 West Allegan, Suite 300
Lansing, MI 48933-1706
(517) 487-1755
(800) 288-5923
www.mpas.org

Minnesota
Minnesota Department of Children,
Families and Learning
Division of Special Education
1500 Highway 36 West
Roseville, MN 55113-4266
(651) 582-8289
cfl.state.mn.us/speced

Rehabilitation Services Branch
Department of Economic Security
390 North Robert St., 5th Floor
St. Paul, MN 55101
(651) 296-1822
www.mnwfc.org

Governor's Council on Developmental
Disabilities
370 Centennial Office Building
658 Cedar St.
St. Paul, MN 55155
(651) 296-4018
www.mncdd.org

Minnesota Disability Law Center
430 First Ave., N., Suite 300
Minneapolis, MN 55401-1780
(312) 332-1441

Mississippi

Office of Special Education
Department of Education
P.O. Box 771
Central High School Building
Jackson, MS 39205-0771
(601) 359-3498
www.mdek12.state.ms.us

Mississippi Office of Vocational
  Rehabilitation
Department of Rehabilitation Services
P.O. Box 1698
Jackson, MS 39215-1698
(601) 853-5230

Developmental Disabilities Planning
  Council
1101 Robert E. Lee Building
239 Lamar St.
Jackson, MS 39210
(601) 359-1288
www.dmh.state.ms.us

Mississippi P&A System
5330 Executive Place, Suite A
Jackson, MS 39206
(601) 981-8207
(800) 772-4057

Missouri

Division of Special Education
Department of Elementary and
  Secondary Education
P.O. Box 480
Jefferson City, MO 65102-0480
(573) 751-5739
www.dese.state.mo.us/divspeced

Division of Vocational Rehabilitation
Department of Education
3024 Dupont Circle
Jefferson City, MO 65109-0525
(573) 751-3251
www.vr.dese.state.mo.us

MO Planning Council for Developmental Disabilities
Division of MR/Developmental
  Disabilities
Department of Mental Health
1706 East Elm
P.O. Box 687
Jefferson City, MO 65102
(573) 751-8611
(800) 500-7878 (in MO)
www.modmh.state.mo.us/mrdd

MO Protection & Advocacy Services
925 South Country Club Drive,
  Unit B-1
Jefferson City, MO 65109
(573) 893-3333
(800) 392-8667

Montana

Special Education Division

Office of Public Instruction

P.O. Box 202501

Helena, MT 59620-2501

(406) 444-4429

Vocational Rehabilitation Program

Department of Public Health and
    Human Services

111 North Sanders St., Room 305

P.O. Box 4210

Helena, MT 59604-4210

(406) 444-2590

Developmental Disabilities Planning
    & Advisory Council

P.O. Box 526

Helena, MT 59624

(406) 444-1334, (800) 337-9942 (in MT)

Montana Advocacy Program

P.O. Box 1680

316 N. Park, Room 211

Helena, MT 59624

(406) 444-3889, (800) 245-4743 (in MT)

Nebraska

Special Populations

Department of Education

P.O. Box 94987

Lincoln, NE 68509-4987

(402) 471-2471

www.edneb.org/SPED/sped.html

Developmental Disabilities Planning
    Council/HHS

P.O. Box 95044

301 Centennial Mall South

Lincoln, NE 68509

(402) 471-2330

www.hhs.state.ne.us

Nebraska Advocacy Services

522 Lincoln Center Building

215 Centennial Mall South

Lincoln, NE 68508

(402) 474-3183

(800) 422-6691

Autism Society of Nebraska

1026 Twin Ridge Road

Lincoln, NE 68510

(402) 423-3796

Nevada

Educational Equity

Department of Education

700 E. Fifth St., Suite 113

Carson City, NV 89701-5096

(775) 687-9171

Rehabilitation Division

Department of Employment, Training
    & Rehabilitation

505 E. King St., Room 502

Carson City, NV 89710

(775) 684-4040

Nevada Disability Advocacy and Law
  Center
6039 Eldora Ave.
Suite C—Box 3
Las Vegas, NV 89146
(702) 257-8150
(888) 349-3843 (toll-free)
www.ndalc.org

New Hampshire
New Hampshire Department of
  Education
78 Regional Drive, Building 2
Concord, NH 03301
(603) 271-3471

New Hampshire Developmental
  Disabilities Council
The Concord Center
10 Ferry St., Unit 315
Concord, NH 03301-5004
(603) 271-3236

Disabilities Rights Center, Inc.
P.O. Box 3660
Concord, NH 03302-3660
(603) 228-0432
(800) 834-1721

Autism Society of New Hampshire
P.O. Box 68
Concord, NH 03302
(603) 898-0916

New Jersey
Office of Special Education Programs
Department of Education
100 Riverview Plaza, P.O. Box 500
Trenton, NJ 08625-0500
(609) 633-6833

Division of Vocational Rehabilitation
  Services
NJ Department of Labor
P.O. Box 398
Trenton, NJ 08625-0398
(609) 292-5987
www.wnjpin.state.nj.us

New Jersey Developmental Disabilities
  Council
20 W. State St., 7th Floor
P.O. Box 700
Trenton, NJ 08625
(609) 292-3745

NJ Protection and Advocacy, Inc.
210 S. Broad St., 3rd Floor
Trenton, NJ 08608
(609) 292-9742
(800) 922-7233 (in NJ)
www.njpanda.org

COSAC (NJ Center for Outreach and
  Services for the Autism Community)
1450 Parkside Ave., Suite 22
Ewing, NJ 08638
(609) 883-8100
Provides information, referral, advocacy,

and parent support for people with
autism, Asperger Syndrome, and
related conditions. Maintains a
national directory of programs.

New Mexico
Special Education
Department of Education
300 Don Gaspar Ave.
Santa Fe, NM 87501-2786
(505) 827-6541
www.sde.state.nm.us

Division of Vocational Rehabilitation
Department of Education
435 St. Michaels Drive, Building D
Santa Fe, NM 87505
(505) 954-8511

New Mexico Developmental Disabilities
    Planning Council
435 St. Michaels Drive, Building D
Santa Fe, NM 87505
(505) 827-7590

Protection and Advocacy System
1720 Louisiana Blvd., NE, Suite 204
Albuquerque, NM 87110
(505) 256-3100
(800) 432-4682 (in NM)

New Mexico Autism Project
2300 Menaul NE
Albuquerque, NM 87107
(505) 272-1852

New York
Office of Vocational and Educational
    Services for Individuals with
    Disabilities
1 Commerce Plaza, Room 1606
Albany, NY 12234
(518) 474-2714
www.nysed.gov

NYS Developmental Disabilities
    Planning Council
155 Washington Ave., 2nd Floor
Albany, NY 12210
(518) 486-7505
(800) 395-3372
www.ddpc.state.ny.us

Autism Advocacy and Outreach
    Group
86 Boyce Ave.
Staten Island, NY 10306
(718) 980-1983

North Carolina
Exceptional Children Division
Department of Public Instruction
301 N. Wilmington St.
Education Building, #670
Raleigh, NC 27601-2825
(919) 715-1565
www.ncgov.com

Child & Adolescent Services
Developmental Disabilities Services
    Section
Division of MH, Disabilities and
    Substance Abuse Services
Department of Health and Human
    Services
3006 Mail Service Center
Raleigh, NC 27699-3006
(919) 733-3654
www.dhhs.state.nc.us

NC Council on Developmental
    Disabilities
1001 Navaho Drive, Suite GL-103
Raleigh, NC 27609
(919) 850-2833
(800) 357-6916
www.nc-ddc.org

Governor's Advisory Council for Persons
    with Disabilities
Bryan Building
2113 Cameron St., Suite 218
Raleigh, NC 27605
(919) 733-9250
(877) 235-4210 (in NC)
www.doa.state.nc.us/dopa/gacpd.htm

Autism Society of North Carolina
505 Oberlin Road, Suite 230
Raleigh, NC 27605-1345
(919) 743-0204
(800) 442-2762

North Dakota
Special Education
Department of Public Instruction
600 E. Boulevard Ave., Dept. 201
Bismarck, ND 58505-0440
(701) 328-2277
www.dpi.state.nd.us/dpi

Disabilities Services Division
ND Department of Human Services
600 S. 2nd St., Suite 1B
Bismarck, ND 58504-5729
(701) 328-8950, (800) 755-2745 (in ND)

North Dakota Developmental
    Disabilities Council
Department of Human Services
600 S. 2nd St., Suite 1B
Bismarck, ND 58504-5729
(701) 328-8953

Protection and Advocacy Project
400 E. Broadway, Suite 409
Bismarck, ND 58501-4071
(701) 328-2950, (800) 472-2670
www.ndcd.org

Northern Mariana Island
Northern Mariana Island Special
    Education
Public School System
P.O. Box 1370 CK
Saipan, MP 96950
(670) 664-3730

Governor's Developmental Disabilities
Council
P.O. Box 2565
Saipan, MP 96950
(670) 322-3014

Northern Mariana's Protection and
Advocacy System
P.O. Box 3529 CK
Saipan, MP 96950
(670) 235-7273

Ohio

Office for Exceptional Children
Ohio Department of Education
25 S. Front St.
Columbus, OH 43215-4104
(614) 466-2650
www.ode.state.oh.us

Rehabilitation Services Commission
400 E. Campus View Blvd.
Columbus, OH 43235-4604
(614) 438-1200
www.state.oh.us/RSC

Ohio Developmental Disabilities
Planning Council
8 E. Long St., Atlas Building,
12th Floor
Columbus, OH 43266-0415
(614) 466-5205
www.state.oh.us/ddc

Ohio Legal Rights Services
8 E. Long St., 5th Floor
Columbus, OH 43215
(614) 466-7264
(800) 282-9181 (in OH)

Oklahoma

Special Education Services
Department of Education
2500 N. Lincoln Blvd.
Oklahoma City, OK 73105-4599
(405) 521-3351

Department of Rehabilitation Services
3535 NW 58th, Suite 500
Oklahoma City, OK 73112
(405) 951-3400

OK Developmental Disabilities
Council
3033 N. Walnut, Suite 105E
P.O. Box 25352
Oklahoma City, OK 73125
(405) 528-4984
(800) 836-4470

Oklahoma Disability Law Center, Inc.
2915 Classen Blvd.
300 Cameron Building
Oklahoma City, OK 73106
(405) 525-7755
(800) 880-7755 (in OK)
www.flash.net/~odlcokc

Oregon

Office of Special Education
Department of Education
255 Capitol St. NE
Salem, OR 97310-0203
(503) 378-3600
www.ode.state.or.us/sped

Vocational Rehabilitation Division
Department of Human Services
500 Summer St., NE
Salem, OR 97310-1018
(503) 945-5880

Oregon Developmental Disabilities
    Council
540 W. 24th Place, NE
Salem, OR 97301-4517
(503) 945-9941
(800) 292-4154 (in OR)
www.oddc.org

Oregon Advocacy Center
620 SW Fifth Ave., 5th Floor
Portland, OR 97204-1428
(503) 243-2081

State Services for Autism
255 Capital St., NE
Salem, OR 97310-0203
(503) 378-3569
www.ode.state.or.us

Autism Society of Oregon
P.O. Box 13884
Salem, OR 97309

Pennsylvania

Bureau of Special Education
Department of Education
333 Market St., 7th Floor
Harrisburg, PA 17126-0333
(717) 783-6913
Special Education Consult Line:
(800) 879-2301

Office of Vocational Rehabilitation
Department of Labor & Industry
1300 Labor & Industry Building
Seventh and Forster St.
Harrisburg, PA 17120
(717) 787-5244
www.dli.state.pa.us

Developmental Disabilities Planning
    Council
561 Forum Building, Commonwealth
    Ave.
Harrisburg, PA 17120
(717) 787-6057

PA Protection and Advocacy, Inc.
116 Pine St.
Harrisburg, PA 17101
(717) 236-8110, (800) 692-7443

Puerto Rico

Assistant Secretary of Special Education
Department of Education
P.O. Box 190759
San Juan, PR 00909-0759
(787) 759-7228

Vocational Rehabilitation Administration
Department of the Family
P.O. Box 191118
San Juan, PR 00919-1118
(787) 729-0160

Puerto Rico Developmental Disabilities
 Council
P.O. Box 9543
San Juan, PR 00908
(787) 722-0595
(787) 725-2333

Office of the Ombudsman for Persons
 with Disabilities
P.O. Box 4234
San Juan, PR 00940-1309
(787) 725-2333

Rhode Island

Office of Special Needs
Department of Education, Shepard
 Building
255 Westminster St., Room 400
Providence, RI 02903-3400
(401) 222-4600

Office of Rehabilitation Services
Department of Human Services
40 Fountain St.
Providence, RI 02903
(401) 421-7005
www.ors.state.ri.us

R.I. Developmental Disabilities Council
14 Harrington Road
Cranston, RI 02920
(401) 737-3395
www.ors.state.ri.us

Rhode Island Disability Law Center
349 Eddy St.
Providence, RI 02903
(401) 831-3150
(800) 733-5332 (in RI)

South Carolina

State Department of Education
Office of Exceptional Children
1429 Senate St., Room 808
Columbia, SC 29201
(803) 734-8806

Vocational Rehabilitation
 Department
1410 Boston Ave., P.O. Box 15
West Columbia, SC 29171-0015
(803) 896-6504

SC Developmental Disabilities Council
1205 Pendleton St., Room 372

Columbia, SC 29201

(803) 734-0456

P&A for People with Disabilities

3710 Landmark Drive, Suite 208

Columbia, SC 29204

(803) 782-0639

(800) 922-5225 (in SC)

South Carolina Autism Society

229 Parson St., Suite A-1

West Columbia, SC 29169

(803) 794-2300

(800) 438-4790

South Dakota

Office of Special Education

700 Governors Drive

Pierre, SD 57501-2291

(605) 773-3678

E-mail: debb@deca.state.sd.us

www.state.sd.us/deca

Division of Rehabilitation Services

Hillsview Plaza, E. Hwy 34

500 E. Capitol

Pierre, SD 57501-5070

(605) 773-3195

www.state.sd.us/dhs/drs

SD Governor's Planning Council on
Developmental Disabilities

Hillsview Plaza, E. Hwy 34

500 E. Capitol

Pierre, SD 57501-5070

(605) 773-6369

www.state.sd.us/dhs/ddc

South Dakota Advocacy Services

221 S. Central Ave.

Pierre, SD 57501

(605) 224-8294

(800) 658-4782 (in SD)

www.sdadvocacy.com

Tennessee

Division of Special Education

Department of Education

Andrew Johnson Tower, 5th Floor

710 James Robertson Parkway

Nashville, TN 37243-0380

(615) 741-2851

www.state.tn.us/education

Division of Rehabilitation Services

Department of Human Services

400 Deaderick St., 15th Floor

Nashville, TN 37248-0060

(615) 313-4714

Tennessee Developmental Disabilities
Council

Cordell Hull Building, 5th Floor

425 Fifth Ave. North

Nashville, TN 37243-0675

(615) 532-6615

Tennessee Protection and Advocacy

P.O. Box 121257

Nashville, TN 37212

(615) 298-1080

(800) 342-1660 (in TN)

Texas

Texas Education Agency
Division of Special Education
1701 N. Congress Ave.
Austin, TX 78701-1494
(512) 463-9414
www.tea.state.tx.us/special.ed

Texas Rehabilitation Commission
4900 N. Lamarr Blvd., Room 7102
Austin, TX 78751-2399
(512) 424-4001

Texas Council for Developmental
   Disabilities
6201 E. Oltorf, Suite 600
Austin, TX 78741
(512) 437-5432
(800) 262-0334
www.rehab.state.tx.us/tpcdd/index/htm
www.txddc.state.tx.us

Advocacy, Inc.
1700 Shoal Creek Blvd.
Austin, TX 78757
(512) 454-4816
(800) 252-9108 (in TX)

Utah

At Risk and Special Education Services
State Office of Education

250 E. 500 South
Salt Lake City, UT 84111-3204
(801) 538-7706

Utah State Office of Rehabilitation
250 E. 500 South
Salt Lake City, UT 84111
(801) 538-7530
www.usor.state.ut.us

Utah Governor's Council for People
   with Disabilities
555 E. 300 South, Suite 201
Salt Lake City, UT 84102
(801) 325-5823
www.gcpd.state.ut.us

Disability Law Center
455 E. 400 South, Suite 410
Salt Lake City, UT 84111
(801) 363-1347
(800) 662-9080 (in UT)
www.disabilitylawcenter.org

Autism Society of Utah
668 S. 1300 East
Salt Lake City, UT 84102
(801) 538-7049

Vermont

Family and Educational Support Team
120 State St., State Office Building
Montpelier, VT 05620-2501
(802) 828-2755

Division of Vocational
    Rehabilitation
Department of Aging & Disabilities
Agency of Human Services
103 S. Main St., Osgood II
Waterbury, VT 05671-2303
(802) 241-2186
www.dad.state.vt.us/dvr/vroffices.htm

Vermont Developmental Disabilities
    Council
103 S. Main St.
Waterbury, VT 05671-0206
(802) 241-2612
(888) 317-2006
www.ahs.state.vt.us/vtddc

Vermont Protection and Advocacy
15 E. State St., #101
Montpelier, VT 05602
(802) 229-1355, (800) 834-7890

Virgin Islands
Special Education/Department of
    Education
44-46 Kongens Gade
Charlotte Amalie
St. Thomas, VI 00802
(340) 774-4399

Division of Disabilities and
    Rehabilitation Services
Knud Hansen Complex, Building A
1303 Hospital Ground
Charlotte Amalie

St. Thomas, VI 00802
(340) 774-0930, ext. 4191

Developmental Disabilities Council
P.O. Box 2671, Kings Hill
St.Croix, VI 00851
(340) 778-9681

Virgin Islands Advocacy Agency
7A Whim, Suite 2
Fredericksted, St. Croix, VI 00840
(340) 772-1200

Virginia
Office of Special Education and Student
    Services
Department of Education
P.O. Box 2120
Richmond, VA 23218-2120
(804) 225-2402
www.pen.k12.va.us

Department of Rehabilitative Services
P.O. Box K300
8004 Franklin Farm Drive
Richmond, VA 23288-0300
(804) 662-7081

Virginia Board for People with
    Disabilities
Ninth Street Office Building
202 N. Ninth St., 9th Floor
Richmond, VA 23219
(804) 786-0016, (800) 846-4464 (in VA)
www.vabord.org

Department for Rights of Virginians
with Disabilities
Ninth Street Office Building, 9th Floor
202 N. Ninth St.
Richmond, VA 23219
(804) 225-2042, (800) 552-3962 (in VA)
www.cns.state.va.us/drvd

Autism Society of America—Peninsula
Chapter
3421 West Lewis Road
Hampton, VA 23666-3830
(757) 827-8226

Washington
Special Education Section
Superintendent of Public Instruction
P.O. Box 47200
Olympia, WA 98504-7200
(360) 725-6075
www.k12.wa.us

Division of Vocational Rehabilitation
Department of Social and Health Services
P.O. Box 4530
Olympia, WA 98504-5340
(360) 438-8008

Developmental Disabilities Council
P.O. Box 48314
Olympia, WA 98504-8314
(360) 753-3908, (800) 634-4473
www.wa.gov/ddc

Autism Society of Washington
203 E. 4th, Suite 507
Olympia, WA 98501
(360) 943-2205

West Virginia
Office of Special Education
Department of Education
1900 Kanahwa Blvd. East
Building 6, Room B-304
Charleston, WV 25305-0330
(304) 558-2696

Division of Rehabilitation Services
State Capitol Complex
P.O. Box 50890
Charleston, WV 25305-0890
(304) 766-4601
www.wvdrs.org

Developmental Disabilities Council
110 Stockton St.
Charleston, WV 25312
(304) 558-0416

Autism Services Center
605 Ninth St.
P.O. Box 507
Huntington, WV 25710-0507
(304) 525-8014

West Virginia Advocates
Litton Building, 4th Floor
1207 Quarrier St.

Charleston, WV 25301

(304) 346-0847, (800) 950-5250 (in WV)

Wisconsin

Division for Learning Support: Equity
and Advocacy

125 S. Webster St.

P.O. Box 7841

Madison, WI 53707-7841

(608) 266-1649, (800) 441-4563

www.dpi.state.wi.us/dpi/dlsea/een

Vocational Rehabilitation

Department of Workforce Development

2917 International Lane, Suite 300

P.O. Box 7852

Madison, WI 53707-7852

(608) 243-5603

www.dwd.state.wi.us/dvr

Wisconsin Council on Developmental
Disabilities

600 Williamshon St.

P.O. Box 7851

Madison, WI 53707-7851

(608) 266-7826

Wisconsin Coalition for Advocacy

16 N. Carroll St., Suite 400

Madison, WI 53703

(608) 267-0214

(800) 928-8778 (in WI)

Autism Society of Wisconsin

103 W. College Ave., Suite 709

Appleton, WI 54911-5744

(920) 993-0279

(888) 4-AUTISM (in WI)

www.asw4autism.org

Wyoming

Department of Education, Special
Programs Unit

Hathaway Building, 2nd Floor

2300 Capitol Ave.

Cheyenne, WY 82002

(307) 777-7389

wydoe.state.wy.us/vocrehab

Division of Vocational Rehabilitation

Department of Employment

1100 Herschler Building

Cheyenne, WY 82002

(307) 777-7389

Governor's Planning Council on
Developmental Disabilities

122 W. 25th St.

Herschler Building

Cheyenne, WY 82002

(307) 777-7115

(800) 442-4333 (in WY)

ddd.state.wy.us

Wyoming P&A System

2424 Pioneer Ave., Suite 101

Cheyenne, WY 82001

(307) 632-3496

(800) 624-7648 (in WY)

Reading List

American Psychiatric Association. *Diagnostic and Statistical Manual of Mental Disorders (DSM-IV)*, 4th ed. Washington, DC: American Psychiatric Association, 1994.

Attwood, Tony. *Asperger's Syndrome: A Guide for Parents and Professionals*. London: Jessica Kingsley Publishers, 1998.

Baker, Bruce L., and Brightman, Alan J. *Steps to Independence: Teaching Everyday Skills to Children with Special Needs*, 3rd ed. Baltimore: Paul H. Brookes, 1997.

Bashe, Patricia Romanowski, and Kirby, Barbara L. *The OASIS Guide to Asperger Syndrome: Advice, Support, Insight and Inspiration*. New York: Crown Publishing, 2001.

Bolick, Teresa. *Asperger Syndrome and Adolescence*. Gloucester, MA: Fair Winds Press, 2001.

Browne, Joy. *Dating for Dummies*. Foster City, CA: IDG Books Worldwide, 1997.

Cohen, D.J., and Volkmar, Fred R., eds. *Handbook of Autism and Pervasive Developmental Disorders*, 2nd ed. New York: John Wiley & Sons, 1997.

Faherty, Catherine. *Asperger's: What Does It Mean to Be Me?* Arlington, TX: Future Horizons, 2000.

Fling, Echo R. *Eating an Artichoke: A Mother's Perspective on Asperger Syndrome.* London and Philadelphia: Jessica Kingsley Publishers, 2000.

Freeman, Sabrina. *Teach Me Language: A Language Manual for Children with Autism, Asperger's Syndrome and Related Developmental Disorders.* Langley, BC: SKF Books, 1997.

Frith, Uta. *Autism: Explaining the Enigma.* Oxford, UK: Basil Blackwell, 1989.

Gale, Linda. *Discover What You're Best At: The National Career Aptitude System and Career Directory*, revised edition. New York: Fireside, 1988.

Grandin, Temple. *Emergence: Labeled Autistic.* Novato, CA: Arena Press, 1986.

Grandin, Temple. *Thinking in Pictures, and Other Reports from My Life with Autism.* New York: Doubleday, 1995.

Greenspan, Stanley, Weidner, Serena, and Simon, Robin, contributor. *The Child with Special Needs: Encouraging Intellectual and Emotional Growth.* New York: Perseus Books, 1998.

Harris, Sandra L. *Siblings of Children with Autism: A Guide for Families.* Bethesda, MD: Woodbine House, 1994.

Howlin, Patricia. *Children with Autism and Asperger Syndrome: A Guide for Practitioners and Carers.* New York: John Wiley & Sons, 1998.

Klin, Ami, Volmar, Fred R., and Sparrow, Sara S., eds. *Asperger Syndrome.* New York: The Guilford Press, 2000.

Kranowitz, Carol Stock. *The Out-of-Sync Child: Recognizing and Coping with Sensory Integration Dysfunction.* New York: Berkley Publishing Group, 1998.

Marsh, Jayne D.B. *From the Heart: On Being the Mother of a Child with Special Needs.* Bethesda, MD: Woodbine House, 1995.

Meyer, Donald, ed. *Uncommon Fathers: Reflections on Raising a Child with a Disability.* Bethesda, MD: Woodbine House, 1995.

Meyer, Donald, ed. *Views from Our Shoes: Growing Up with a Brother or Sister with Special Needs.* Bethesda, MD: Woodbine House, 1997.

Meyer, Donald, Vadasy, Patricia, and Fewell, Rebecca. *Living with a Brother or Sister with Special Needs: A Book for Sibs,* 2nd ed. Seattle: University of Washington Press, 1996.

Murphy, Kevin. *Out of the Fog: Treatment Options and Coping Strategies for Adult Attention Deficit Disorder.* New York: Hyperion, 1995.

Myles, Brenda Smith, and Simpson, Richard L. *Asperger Syndrome: A Guide for Educators and Parents.* Austin, TX: Pro-Ed, 1998.

Myles, Brenda Smith, and Southwick, Jack. *Asperger Syndrome and Difficult Moments: Practical Solutions for Tantrums, Rage, and Meltdowns.* Shawnee Mission, KS: Autism Asperger Publishing Co., 1999.

Poland, Janet. *The Sensitive Child.* New York: St. Martin's Press, 1995.

Powers, Michael D., ed. *Children with Autism: A Parent's Guide,* 2nd ed. Bethesda, MD: Woodbine House, 2000.

Ratey, John J., and Johnson, Catherine. *Shadow Syndromes: The Mild Forms of Major Mental Disorders That Sabotage Us.* New York: Bantam Books, 1997.

Schopler, Eric, ed. *Parent Survival Manual: A Guide to Crisis Resolution in Autism and Related Developmental Disorders.* New York: Plenum Books, 1995.

Schultz, Robert T., Romanski, Lizabeth M., and Tsatsanis, Katherine D., "Neurofunctional Models of Autistic Disorder and Asperger Syndrome: Clues from Neuroimaging," in Klin, Ami, Volkmar, Fred R., and Sparrow, Sara S., eds. *Asperger Syndrome.* New York: The Guilford Press, 2000.

Siegel, Lawrence. *The Complete IEP Guide: How to Advocate for Your Special Ed Child.* Berkeley, CA: Nolo.com, 1999.

Stengle, Linda. *Laying Community Foundations for Your Child with a Disability: How to Establish Relationships that Will Support Your Child After You're Gone.* Bethesda, MD: Woodbine House, 1996.

Twachtman-Cullen, Diane. *How to Be a Para-Pro.* Higganum, CT: Starfish Specialty Press, 2000.

Willey, Liane. *Pretending to Be Normal: Living with Asperger's Syndrome.* London: Jessica Kingsley Publishers, 1999.

Wing, Lorna. *The Autistic Spectrum: A Parent's Guide to Understanding and Helping Your Child.* Ulysses Press, 2001.

Bibliography

Chapter One

American Psychiatric Association, *Diagnostic and Statistical Manual of Mental Disorders (DSM-IV)*, 4th ed. Washington, DC: American Psychiatric Association, 1994.

Asperger's Syndrome Association of New England, *Disclosure and Asperger's Syndrome: Our Own Stories*, Newton, MA, 2000.

Attwood, Tony. *Asperger's Syndrome: A Guide for Parents and Professionals*. London: Jessica Kingsley Publishers, 1998.

Faherty, Catherine. *Asperger's: What Does It Mean to Be Me?: A Workbook Explaining Self-Awareness and Life Lessons to the Child or Youth with High-Functioning Autism or Asperger's*. Arlington, TX: Future Horizons, 2000.

Gray, Carol. "Pictures of Me: Introducing Students with Asperger Syndrome to Their Talents, Personalities, and Diagnosis," from *The Morning News*, Jenison, Mich: Jenison Public Schools, Fall 1996.

Harris, Sandra L. "Your Child's Development," in Powers, Michael D., ed. *Children with Autism: A Parent's Guide*, 2nd ed. Bethesda, MD: Woodbine House, 2000.

Klin, Ami, and Volkmar, Fred R. "Diagnostic Issues in Asperger Syndrome," in Klin, Ami, Volkmar, Fred R., and Sparrow, Sara S., eds. *Asperger Syndrome*. New York: The Guilford Press, 2000.

Myles, Brenda Smith, and Simpson, Richard L. *Asperger Syndrome: A Guide for Educators and Parents*. Austin, TX: Pro-Ed, 1998.

Ozonoff, Sally, and Griffith, Elizabeth McMahon. "Neuropsychological Function and the External Validity of Asperger Syndrome," in Klin, Ami, Volkmar, Fred R., and Sparrow, Sara S., eds. *Asperger Syndrome*. New York: The Guilford Press, 2000.

Powers, Michael D. "What Is Autism?" in Powers, Michael D., ed. *Children with Autism: A Parent's Guide*, 2nd ed. Bethesda, MD: Woodbine House, 2000.

Vermeulen, Peter. *I Am Special: Introducing Children and Young People to Their Autistic Spectrum Disorder*. London and Philadelphia: Jessica Kingsley Publishers, 2000.

Chapter Two

Baron-Cohen, Simon. *Mindblindness: An Essay on Autism and Theory of Mind*. Cambridge: MIT Press, 1995.

Frith, Uta. *Autism: Explaining the Enigma*. Oxford, UK: Basil Blackwell, 1989.

Ratey, John J., and Johnson, Catherine. *Shadow Syndromes: The Mild Forms of Major Mental Disorders That Sabotage Us*. New York: Bantam Books, 1997.

Schultz, Robert T., Romanski, Lizabeth M., and Tsatsanis, Katherine D., "Neurofunctional Models of Autistic Disorder and Asperger Syndrome: Clues from Neuroimaging," in Klin, Ami, Volkmar, Fred R., and Sparrow, Sara S., eds. *Asperger Syndrome*. New York: The Guilford Press, 2000.

Volkmar, Fred R., "Medical Problems, Treatments, and Professionals," in Powers, Michael D., ed. *Children with Autism: A Parent's Guide*, 2nd ed. Bethesda, MD: Woodbine House, 2000.

Wing, Lorna. *Asperger Syndrome: A Clinical Account*. Psychological Medicine, 1981.

Chapter Three

Folstein, Susan E., and Santangelo, Susan L., "Does Asperger Syndrome Aggregate in Families?" in Klin, Ami, Volkmar, Fred R., and Sparrow, Sara S., eds. *Asperger Syndrome*. New York: The Guilford Press, 2000.

Klin, Ami, and Volkmar, Fred R., "Diagnostic Issues in Asperger Syndrome," in Klin, Ami, Volkmar, Fred R., and Sparrow, Sara S., eds. *Asperger Syndrome*. New York: The Guilford Press, 2000.

Martin, Andres, Patzer, David K., and Volkmar, Fred R., "Psychopharmacological Treatment of Higher-Functioning Pervasive Developmental Disorders," in Klin, Ami, Volkmar, Fred R., and Sparrow, Sara S., eds. *Asperger Syndrome*. New York: The Guilford Press, 2000.

Tommasone, Lillian and Joe. "Adjusting to Your Child's Diagnosis," in Powers, Michael D., ed. *Children with Autism: A Parent's Guide,* 2nd ed. Bethesda, MD: Woodbine House, 2000.

Wilens, Timothy. *Straight Talk About Psychiatric Medications for Kids*. New York: The Guilford Press, 1999.

Chapter Four
Baron-Cohen, Simon. *Mindblindness: An Essay on Autism and Theory of Mind*. Cambridge: MIT Press, 1995.

Grandin, Temple. *Thinking in Pictures, and Other Reports from My Life with Autism*. New York: Doubleday, 1995.

Grandin, Temple. *Emergence: Labeled Autistic*. Novato, CA: Arena Press, 1986.

Kranowitz, Carol Stock. *The Out-of-Sync Child: Recognizing and Coping with Sensory Integration Dysfunction*. New York: Berkley Publishing Group, 1998.

Poland, Janet. *The Sensitive Child*. New York: St. Martin's Press, 1995.

Williams, Donna. *Nobody Nowhere: The Extraordinary Autobiography of an Autistic*. New York: Avon Books, 1994.

Williams, Donna. *Somebody Somewhere: Breaking Free from the World of Autism*. New York: Times Books, 1995.

Chapter Five
Bruey, Carolyn Thorwarth. "Daily Life with Your Child," in Powers, Michael D., ed. *Children with Autism: A Parent's Guide,* 2nd ed. Bethesda, MD: Woodbine House, 2000.

Ozonoff, Sally, and Griffith, Elizabeth McMahon. "Neuropsychological Function and the External Validity of Asperger Syndrome," in Klin, Ami, Volkmar, Fred R., and Sparrow, Sara S., eds. *Asperger Syndrome*. New York: The Guilford Press, 2000.

Powers, Michael D. "Children with Autism and Their Families," in Powers, Michael D., ed. *Children with Autism: A Parent's Guide,* 2nd ed. Bethesda, MD: Woodbine House, 2000.

Willey, Liane Holliday. *Asperger Syndrome in the Family: Redefining Normal.* London and Philadelphia: Jessica Kingsley Publishers, 2001.

Willey, Liane Holliday. *Pretending to be Normal.* London and Philadelphia: Jessica Kingsley Publishers, 1999.

Williams, Donna. *Nobody Nowhere: The Extraordinary Autobiography of an Autistic.* New York: Avon Books, 1994.

Williams, Donna. *Somebody Somewhere: Breaking Free from the World of Autism.* New York: Times Books, 1995.

Chapter Six

Powers, Michael D., ed. *Children with Autism: A Parent's Guide,* 2nd ed. Bethesda, MD: Woodbine House, 2000.

Goldstein, Arnold P., and McGinnis, Ellen. *Skillstreaming in Early Childhood: Teaching Prosocial Skills to the Preschool and Kindergarten Child.* Champaign, IL: Research Press, 1990.

Gray, Carol. *New Social Stories.* Arlington, TX: Future Horizons, 2000.

Chapter Seven

Egel, Andrew L. "Finding the Right Early Intervention and Educational Programs," in Powers, Michael D., ed. *Children with Autism: A Parent's Guide,* 2nd ed. Bethesda, MD: Woodbine House, 2000.

Fouse, Beth. *Creating a "Win-Win IEP" for Students with Autism.* Arlington, TX: Future Horizons, 1999.

Friedlander, Bernice. "Becoming an Advocate," in Powers, Michael D., ed. *Children with Autism: A Parent's Guide,* 2nd ed. Bethesda, MD: Woodbine House, 2000.

Goldstein, Arnold, and McGinnis, Ellen. *Skillstreaming the Elementary School Child: New Strategies and Perspectives for Teaching Prosocial Skills.* Champaign, IL: Research Press, 1997.

Kaplan, James E., and Moore, Ralph J. Jr. "Legal Rights and Hurdles," in Powers, Michael D., ed. *Children with Autism: A Parent's Guide,* 2nd ed. Bethesda, MD: Woodbine House, 2000.

Klin, Ami, et al. "Assessment Issues in Children and Adolescents with Asperger Syndrome," in Klin, Ami, Volkmar, Fred R., and Sparrow, Sara S., eds. *Asperger Syndrome*. New York: The Guilford Press, 2000.

Klin, Ami, and Volkmar, Fred R. "Treatment and Intervention Guidelines for Individuals with Asperger Syndrome," in Klin, Ami, Volkmar, Fred R., and Sparrow, Sara S., eds. *Asperger Syndrome*. New York: The Guilford Press, 2000.

Moreno, Susan, and O'Neal, Carol. "Tips for Teaching High-Functioning People with Autism." Crown Point, IN: MAAP Services, Inc.

Myles, Brenda Smith, and Simpson, Richard L. *Asperger Syndrome: A Guide for Educators and Parents*. Austin, TX: Pro-Ed, 1998.

Rourke, Byron P., and Tsatsanis, Katherine D. "Nonverbal Learning Disabilities and Asperger Syndrome," in Klin, Ami, Volkmar, Fred R., and Sparrow, Sara S., eds., *Asperger Syndrome*. New York: The Guilford Press, 2000.

Tanguay, Pamela B. *Nonverbal Learning Disabilities at Home: A Parent's Guide*. London and Philadelphia: Jessica Kingsley Publishers, 2001.

Thompson, Sue. *The Source for Nonverbal Learning Disorders*. East Moline, IL: LinguiSystems, 1997.

Twachtman-Cullen, Diane. *How to Be a Para Pro: A Comprehensive Training Manual for Paraprofessionals*. Higganum, CT: Starfish Specialty Press, 2000.

Williams, Karen. "Understanding the Student with Asperger Syndrome: Guidelines for Teachers," *Focus on Autistic Behavior*, vol. 10, no. 2, June, 1995.

Wright, Peter W.D., and Wright, Pamela Darr. *Wrightslaw: Special Education Law*. Hartfield, VA: Harbor House Law Press, 1999.

Chapter Eight

Baker, Jed. *Social Skills Training for Children with Asperger Syndrome, High-Functioning Autism, and Related Social Communication Disorders: A Manual for Practitioners*. Shawnee Mission, KS: Autism Asperger Publishing Co., 2002.

Gray, Carol. *New Social Stories*. Arlington, TX: Future Horizons, 2000.

Gray, Carol. *Comic Strip Conversations*. Arlington, TX: Future Horizons, 1994.

Freeman, Sabrina, and Dake, Lorelei. *Teach Me Language: A Language Manual for Children with Autism, Asperger Syndrome, and Related Developmental Disorders*. Langley, B.C.: SKF Books, 1997; and *The Companion Exercise Forms for Teach Me Language*. Langley, B.C.: SKF Books, 1997.

Howlin, Patricia, Baron-Cohen, Simon, and Hadwin, Julie. *Teaching Children with Autism to Mind-Read: A Practical Guide*. Chichester, England: John Wiley & Sons, 1999.

Klin, Ami, et al. "Assessment Issues in Children and Adolescents with Asperger Syndrome," in Klin, Ami, Volkmar, Fred R., and Sparrow, Sara S., eds. *Asperger Syndrome*. New York: The Guilford Press, 2000.

Klin, Ami, and Volkmar, Fred R. "Treatment and Intervention Guidelines for Individuals with Asperger Syndrome," in Klin, Ami, Volkmar, Fred R., and Sparrow, Sara S., eds. *Asperger Syndrome*. New York: The Guilford Press, 2000.

La Voie, Richard, in Bieber, J. (producer), "Learning Disabilities and Social Skills," Washington, DC: Public Broadcasting Service, 1994.

Rourke, Byron P., and Tsatsanis, Katherine D. "Nonverbal Learning Disabilities and Asperger Syndrome," in Klin, Ami, Volkmar, Fred R., and Sparrow, Sara S., eds. *Asperger Syndrome*. New York: The Guilford Press, 2000.

Savner, Jennifer L., and Myles, Brenda Smith. *Making Visual Supports Work in the Home and Community: Strategies for Individuals with Autism and Asperger Syndrome*. Shawnee Mission, KS: Autism Asperger Publishing, 2000.

Tanguay, Pamela B. *Nonverbal Learning Disabilities at Home: A Parent's Guide*. London and Philadelphia: Jessica Kingsley Publishers, 2001.

Thompson, Sue. *The Source for Nonverbal Learning Disorders*. East Moline, IL: LinguiSystems, 1997.

Twachtman-Cullen, Diane. *How to Be a Para Pro: A Comprehensive Training Manual for Paraprofessionals*. Higganum, CT: Starfish Specialty Press, 2000.

Chapter Nine

Bolick, Teresa. *Asperger Syndrome and Adolescence: Helping Preteens and Teens Get Ready for the Real World.* Gloucester, MA: Fair Winds Press, 2001.

Brown, Joy. *Dating for Dummies.* Foster City, CA: IDG Books Worldwide, 1977.

Goldstein, Arnold, and McGinnis, Ellen. *Skillstreaming the Adolescent.* Champaign, IL: Research Press, 1997.

Koplewicz, Harold S. *Depression in Children and Adolescents.* New York: Harwood Academic Publications, 1992.

Meyer, Roger N. *Asperger Syndrome Employment Workbook: An Employment Workbook for Adults with Asperger Syndrome.* London and Philadelphia: Jessica Kingsley Publishers, 2001.

Tantam, Digby. "Adolescence and Adulthood of Individuals with Asperger Syndrome," in Klin, Ami, Volkmar, Fred R., and Sparrow, Sara S., eds. *Asperger Syndrome.* New York: The Guilford Press, 2000.

Chapter Ten

Attwood, Tony. *Asperger's Syndrome: A Guide for Parents and Professionals.* London: Jessica Kingsley Publishers, 1998.

Holmes, David L. "The Years Ahead: Adults with Autism," in Powers, Michael D., ed. *Children with Autism: A Parent's Guide,* 2nd ed. Bethesda, MD: Woodbine House, 2000.

Klin, Ami, et al. "Assessment Issues in Children and Adolescents with Asperger Syndrome," in Klin, Ami, Sparrow, Sara S., and Volkmar, Fred R., eds. *Asperger Syndrome.* New York: The Guilford Press, 2000.

Leaf, Ronald, and McEachin, John, eds. *Work in Progress.* New York: DRL Books, LLC, 1999.

Meyer, Roger N. *Asperger Syndrome Employment Workbook: An Employment Workbook for Adults with Asperger Syndrome.* London and Philadelphia: Jessica Kingsley Publishers, 2001.

Newport, Jerry. "The Letter I Never Wrote to My Parents," *Autism/Asperger Digest,* Future Horizons, May-June, 2000.

Tantam, Digby. "Adolescence and Adulthood of Individuals with Asperger Syndrome," in Klin, Ami, Volkmar, Fred R., and Sparrow, Sara S., eds. *Asperger Syndrome*. New York: The Guilford Press, 2000.

Williams, Donna. *Nobody Nowhere: The Extraordinary Autobiography of an Autistic*. New York: Avon Books, 1994.

Williams, Donna. *Somebody Somewhere: Breaking Free from the World of Autism*. New York: Times Books, 1995.

Index